Finally, It All Makes Sense

The Complete Late Diagnosis Autism Guide for Women

Schmidt Annette Mattisson

ISBN: 978-1-7641438-5-1

First Edition: 2025

Isohan Publishing

This book is for informational and educational purposes only. The content is not intended to be a substitute for professional medical advice, diagnosis, or treatment. Always seek the advice of your physician or other qualified health provider with any questions you may have regarding a medical condition or mental health concern.

The author and publisher make no representations or warranties about the accuracy, completeness, or suitability of the information contained in this book. The information provided is based on research, professional experience, and personal accounts, but individual experiences may vary.

The assessment tools, checklists, and strategies presented in this book are not diagnostic instruments and should not be used as substitutes for professional evaluation by qualified healthcare providers.

The names and scenarios depicted in this book are purely for illustrative purposes only. Any resemblance to actual

Readers are encouraged to seek professional support from healthcare providers, therapists, and other qualified professionals familiar with autism spectrum conditions when making important decisions about diagnosis, treatment, or life changes.

Table of Contents

Chapter 1: The Missing Pieces

- Recognizing Autism in Adult Women

The medical textbooks got it wrong. For decades, autism research focused almost exclusively on boys—specifically, white boys who displayed obvious repetitive behaviors and struggled with verbal communication. This narrow lens left millions of women undiagnosed, misunderstood, and questioning their place in the world (1). You might be one of them.

Sarah, a 34-year-old marketing manager, spent years thinking she was broken. She could deliver flawless presentations but felt completely drained after team meetings. She organized her closet by color and texture, a habit that seemed quirky until she realized how distressed she became when things were out of place. She had one close friend but struggled to maintain casual acquaintanceships. Sarah's story isn't unique—it's the story of countless women who've learned to hide their authentic selves so well that even they forgot who they really were.

The Great Masquerade

Women with autism become master actors without ever auditioning for the role. From childhood, girls receive different social messages than boys. While a boy might be labeled "quirky" or "intense," a girl displaying similar traits gets corrected, redirected, or taught to "be more like the other girls" (2). This societal pressure creates what researchers call masking—the conscious or unconscious suppression of autistic traits to appear neurotypical.

Dr. Michelle Mowery's research shows that girls learn to camouflage their differences through careful observation and mimicry (3). They study social interactions like scientists, creating internal scripts for different situations. A woman might rehearse casual conversations in her head, practice facial expressions in the mirror, or force herself to make eye contact despite the discomfort it causes.

Consider Maria, a 29-year-old teacher who developed an elaborate system for social navigation. She created mental categories for different types of small talk, memorized appropriate responses to common questions, and even practiced her laugh to sound more natural. She was so successful at this performance that colleagues described her as outgoing and social. Inside, Maria felt like she was watching her life through a window—present but disconnected.

The Textbook Trap

Traditional autism criteria were built around male presentations, creating a diagnostic blind spot for women (4). The stereotypical image of autism—a child who rocks back and forth, avoids eye contact, and speaks in a monotone—captures only a fraction of the autistic experience. Women often present differently, displaying what researchers call "internalized" rather than "externalized" behaviors.

Take stimming, for example. Boys might flap their hands or spin objects, behaviors that are visible and easily identified. Women are more likely to engage in subtle stimming: twirling their hair, picking at their skin, or tapping their fingers in patterns. These behaviors often go unnoticed or get dismissed as nervous habits (5).

The intensity of interests also manifests differently. While boys might obsess over trains or dinosaurs—interests that stand out as unusual—girls often develop intense interests in socially acceptable topics like horses, books, or celebrities. Lisa, now 38, spent her childhood memorizing every detail about her favorite pop stars. She could recite discographies, tour dates, and personal histories with encyclopedic accuracy. Her parents saw this as typical teenage behavior, not recognizing it as a special interest.

The Little Professor Meets the Good Girl

Autism in women often splits into two primary presentations: the "little professor" and the "good girl." Understanding these patterns can help you recognize autism in yourself or others (6).

The Little Professor displays obvious intelligence and speaks with advanced vocabulary, often appearing mature beyond her years. She might correct adults' grammar, share lengthy explanations about her interests, or struggle with age-appropriate social expectations. Jessica, now 42, remembers being called "an old soul" throughout childhood. She preferred reading to playing with dolls and could discuss complex topics with adults while struggling to connect with peers her own age.

The Good Girl flies under the radar entirely. She follows rules meticulously, rarely causes problems, and appears to adapt well to social situations. Teachers and parents praise her compliance, missing the internal struggle she faces. Rachel, a 35-year-old nurse, was the perfect student—quiet, attentive, and never disruptive. She followed social rules so carefully that no one noticed her difficulty reading social cues or her exhaustion from constant vigilance.

Both presentations share common threads: intense internal experiences, difficulty with unwritten social rules, and a sense of being different from peers. The key difference lies in how these traits manifest externally and how others respond to them (7).

Red Flags That Point to Autism

Recognizing autism in adult women requires looking beyond stereotypes to identify subtle but consistent patterns. These red flags often appear across multiple life domains and persist over time.

Sensory overwhelm represents one of the most reliable indicators. You might find yourself covering your ears in restaurants, cutting tags out of clothing, or feeling physically ill in fluorescent lighting. Amanda, a 31-year-old graphic designer, thought everyone felt nauseous in grocery stores until she realized the combination of sounds, smells, and visual stimulation affected her more intensely than others.

Social exhaustion after seemingly normal interactions signals another red flag. If you need hours or days to recover from social events, experience relief when plans get cancelled, or feel like you're performing rather than connecting, you might be experiencing autistic burnout (8). This exhaustion stems from the cognitive load required to navigate neurotypical social expectations.

Intense interests that consume your attention and energy, even if they seem socially acceptable, can indicate autism. These interests provide joy, comfort, and expertise but might interfere with other activities or relationships. Dr. Patricia Howlin's research identifies this pattern as a core feature of autism, regardless of the specific interest topic (9).

Executive function challenges often appear as difficulty with transitions, time management, or task initiation. You might excel in structured environments but struggle when routines change unexpectedly. Caroline, a 40-year-old accountant, thrived during tax season's predictable demands but felt paralyzed when asked to take on new projects without clear guidelines.

Self-Assessment Tools and Reflection

Several validated screening tools can help identify autistic traits in adult women, though they're not substitutes for professional diagnosis. The Autism Spectrum Quotient (AQ) provides a starting point, with scores above 32 suggesting further evaluation may be warranted (10). The Camouflaging Autistic Traits Questionnaire (CAT-Q) specifically measures masking behaviors common in women (11).

More than formal assessments, personal reflection often provides the clearest insights. Consider these questions:

- Do you feel like you're acting or performing in social situations?

- Have you developed elaborate systems or rules for social interaction?

- Do you experience physical exhaustion after social events?

- Are there specific textures, sounds, or environments that cause you distress?

- Do you have interests that others consider unusual in their intensity or focus?

- Have you always felt slightly "different" from your peers without being able to identify why?

Keep a sensory and energy journal for two weeks. Note situations that drain or energize you, physical reactions to environments, and social interactions that feel particularly challenging or effortless. Patterns often emerge that point toward autistic traits.

Recognition Stories from Real Women

Understanding autism in women becomes clearer through real experiences. These stories illustrate the diverse ways autism can manifest and the relief that comes with recognition.

Elena's Story: At 28, Elena was a successful software engineer who struggled with office politics and team dynamics. She excelled at coding but felt lost during casual conversations and group meetings. After reading about autism in women online, she recognized her childhood pattern of intense interests (she memorized entire books about marine biology), her need for routine, and her sensory sensitivities. The diagnosis at 29 explained decades of feeling like an outsider in her own life.

Patricia's Story: Patricia didn't consider autism until her daughter was diagnosed at age 8. Researching autism to support her child, Patricia recognized her own traits: the way she organized her closet by color and season, her difficulty making casual friends, and her need for detailed plans before any social event. At 45, she realized that what she'd called "high standards" and "introversion" were actually autistic traits that had shaped her entire life.

Monica's Story: Monica, now 52, spent years in therapy for anxiety and depression before a therapist suggested autism evaluation. She'd always been the "responsible one" in her family, following rules perfectly and avoiding conflict. Her autism diagnosis reframed her childhood experiences: her intense love of reading wasn't just being studious, her difficulty with surprise visits wasn't just shyness, and her need for alone time wasn't antisocial behavior.

Each woman's recognition journey was different, but all shared common elements: a sense of finally understanding themselves, relief at having an explanation for lifelong differences, and sometimes grief for the years spent trying to be someone they weren't.

Moving Forward with Recognition

Recognizing autism in yourself doesn't require immediate action or disclosure. This recognition is yours to process, explore, and act upon in whatever way feels right for you. Some women pursue formal diagnosis, while others find that understanding their autistic traits is sufficient for personal growth and self-acceptance.

What matters most is approaching this recognition with curiosity rather than judgment. Autism isn't something to fix or cure—it's a neurological difference that influences how you experience and interact with the world (12). This difference has likely contributed to your unique strengths, perspectives, and abilities, even as it may have created challenges in a world designed for neurotypical brains.

The women who shared their stories all emphasized one crucial point: recognizing their autism didn't change who they were, but it changed how they understood themselves.

This understanding opened doors to better self-advocacy, more authentic relationships, and strategies that actually worked with their brains rather than against them.

Wrapping Up the Recognition Process

Recognition marks the beginning of a journey, not the end of a search. You now have language for experiences that may have felt confusing or isolating. You understand that the differences you've always sensed in yourself have a name and a community of others who share similar experiences.

This recognition process takes time. Be patient with yourself as you process this information and consider what it means for your life moving forward. The next step involves deciding what to do with this recognition—whether that means seeking professional diagnosis, connecting with autistic communities, or simply using this knowledge to better understand and care for yourself.

Chapter 2: The Diagnostic Journey

- Navigating Professional Assessment

Getting an autism diagnosis as an adult woman often feels like solving a puzzle with missing pieces. The healthcare system wasn't designed with you in mind, and finding professionals who understand how autism presents in women requires persistence, research, and sometimes a bit of luck. This journey can be frustrating, but it's also empowering when you find the right support.

Dr. Sarah Hendrickx, an autism specialist, notes that women seeking diagnosis often arrive with decades of masking and adaptation, making their autistic traits less obvious to clinicians trained to recognize male presentations (13). This reality means you'll need to advocate for yourself throughout the process, armed with knowledge about what to expect and how to prepare.

Finding Qualified Diagnosticians

Not all mental health professionals understand autism in women. You need someone specifically trained in autism assessment who recognizes female presentations and understands the masking phenomenon. This specialist knowledge makes the difference between accurate diagnosis and years of continued confusion.

Start your search with autism organizations in your area. The Autism Society and local autism support groups often maintain lists of recommended diagnosticians. Online autism communities, particularly those focused on women and late diagnosis, can provide valuable recommendations based on personal experiences (14).

Research potential providers thoroughly. Look for psychologists, psychiatrists, or developmental pediatricians (some see adults) who specifically mention autism assessment in women on their websites. Check their credentials and experience. Dr. Amanda Richdale's research emphasizes the importance of clinicians who understand the unique presentation patterns in women (15).

Ask potential providers specific questions during initial consultations:

- How many adult women have you diagnosed with autism?

- Are you familiar with masking and camouflaging behaviors?

- What assessment tools do you use for adult women?

- How long is your assessment process?

- Do you understand how autism can co-occur with other conditions common in women?

Red flags include providers who dismiss your concerns because you made eye contact, seem "too social," or don't fit stereotypical autism presentations. Trust your instincts— if a provider doesn't seem to understand your experience, continue your search.

Consider specialized autism clinics if they're available in your area. These centers often have teams trained specifically in autism assessment and understand the nuances of adult diagnosis. While they may have longer waiting lists, the expertise can be worth the wait.

Telehealth options have expanded access to qualified providers. Some specialists offer remote assessments, particularly helpful if you live in an area with limited local resources. Ensure any telehealth provider is licensed in your state and follows proper assessment protocols.

What to Expect During Assessment

Autism assessment typically involves multiple appointments and various evaluation methods. Understanding this process helps reduce anxiety and ensures you're prepared to provide necessary information.

Initial consultation usually lasts 1-2 hours and involves discussing your concerns, medical history, and current challenges. The provider will ask about your childhood, development, and current functioning across different life areas. This conversation helps determine if formal assessment is appropriate.

Psychological testing forms the core of most assessments. The Autism Diagnostic Observation Schedule (ADOS-2) remains the gold standard, though it wasn't originally designed for adult women and may miss subtle presentations (16). Some providers supplement with tools specifically designed for women, such as the Girls Questionnaire (GQ) or focus on detailed clinical interviews.

During testing, you'll engage in various activities while the provider observes your communication style, social interaction patterns, and behavioral responses. Don't try to mask or perform during these sessions—the goal is to see your natural responses and communication style.

Developmental history requires detailed information about your childhood. Many women struggle with this aspect because they masked effectively or received messages that their behaviors were "wrong" and needed changing. Gather whatever information you can from family members, school records, or childhood friends.

Collateral information from family members or close friends can provide valuable perspective on your traits and behaviors. Some providers request interviews with people who've known you since childhood or can observe your unmasked behaviors.

The process timeline varies significantly. Some providers complete assessments in one day, while others spread it across multiple appointments over several weeks. Prepare for the possibility that you might need to wait between appointments or for results.

Preparing for Your Evaluation

Thorough preparation significantly improves your assessment experience and ensures the provider gets accurate information about your autistic traits. This preparation is particularly important for women who've become skilled at masking.

Document your experiences in detail before the assessment. Create lists of sensory sensitivities, social challenges, special interests, and repetitive behaviors. Include examples from childhood and adulthood. Sarah, a 36-year-old teacher, created a detailed timeline of her traits across different life stages, helping her provider understand the consistency of her autistic characteristics.

Gather childhood evidence whenever possible. School reports, report cards, baby books, or family photos can provide valuable information about early development. Look for comments about being "mature for your age," "a perfectionist," "shy," or "in her own world." These seemingly positive descriptions often indicate masked autism in girls.

Create a sensory profile by documenting your reactions to different environments, textures, sounds, and visual stimuli. Note both sensitivities (things that overwhelm you) and seeking behaviors (things you crave or find calming). Include strategies you've developed to manage sensory challenges.

List your special interests throughout your life, even if they seem "normal" for girls. Include the intensity and duration of these interests, how they affected your daily life, and any expertise you developed. Dr. Francesca Happé's research shows that special interests in women often focus on socially acceptable topics, making them easy to overlook (17).

Bring examples of masking and camouflaging behaviors. Describe situations where you felt like you were acting or performing, scripts you've developed for social situations, or times when you studied others to learn appropriate behaviors. This information helps providers understand the effort you've put into appearing neurotypical.

Prepare for emotional reactions during the assessment. Many women feel vulnerable discussing lifelong struggles or relieved to finally have their experiences taken seriously. It's normal to feel emotionally overwhelmed during or after sessions.

Understanding Diagnostic Criteria and Limitations

Current diagnostic criteria in the DSM-5 still reflect male-biased research, creating challenges for women seeking accurate diagnosis. Understanding these limitations helps you advocate for yourself and interpret results appropriately.

The DSM-5 criteria focus on observable behaviors rather than internal experiences, potentially missing the subtle ways autism manifests in women. The criteria emphasize repetitive behaviors that are obvious rather than internalized, social communication challenges that may be masked, and sensory differences that women often manage privately (18).

Research limitations affect how providers understand autism in women. Most autism research historically focused on boys and men, creating a knowledge gap about female presentations. Dr. Eileen Lai's work highlights how this bias leads to underdiagnosis in women and girls (19).

Masking compensation can make autistic traits less visible during assessment. If you've spent decades learning to appear neurotypical, you might automatically mask during evaluation sessions. Discuss this tendency with your provider and consider bringing someone who's seen your unmasked behaviors.

Co-occurring conditions common in autistic women can complicate diagnosis. Anxiety, depression, eating disorders, and ADHD often develop as responses to undiagnosed autism but might overshadow underlying autistic traits. Experienced providers understand these connections and assess for autism even when other conditions are present (20).

Cultural factors can influence how autism presents and how symptoms are interpreted. Different cultural backgrounds may have varying expectations for social behavior, expression of distress, or gender roles that affect assessment results.

Private vs. Public Healthcare Pathways

The choice between private and public healthcare options affects your diagnostic experience, timeline, and costs. Each pathway has distinct advantages and challenges that influence your decision.

Private healthcare typically offers shorter wait times and more personalized service. Private providers often have more time for thorough assessments and may be more familiar with autism in women. You can choose your provider based on their expertise and approach rather than being assigned to available professionals.

Private assessment allows for more flexibility in scheduling and often includes detailed written reports that you own and can share as needed. The relationship with your provider may continue beyond diagnosis, offering ongoing support and recommendations.

However, private assessment costs can be significant, ranging from $1,500 to $5,000 depending on your location and the provider's approach. Insurance coverage varies widely, with many plans excluding autism assessment for adults or requiring substantial documentation of medical necessity.

Public healthcare pathways through community mental health centers or public hospitals may offer free or low-cost assessment but often involve longer wait times. The providers may have less experience with adult autism, particularly in women, and appointments might feel rushed due to time constraints.

Public systems sometimes focus on determining eligibility for services rather than providing comprehensive understanding of your autistic traits. The assessment might be more limited in scope, potentially missing subtle presentations common in women.

Insurance considerations significantly impact your options. Contact your insurance provider to understand coverage for autism assessment in adults. Some plans cover assessment if it's deemed medically necessary, while others exclude it entirely. Get pre-authorization in writing when possible to avoid unexpected bills.

Cost Considerations and Financial Planning

Autism assessment represents a significant financial investment, but planning and research can help manage costs and identify funding options.

Assessment costs vary widely based on location, provider experience, and assessment scope. Basic assessments might cost $1,500-$2,500, while thorough evaluations can reach $5,000 or more. Factor in potential travel costs if qualified providers aren't available locally.

Insurance navigation requires patience and persistence. Call your insurance company to ask specifically about autism assessment coverage for adults. Request written documentation of your benefits and any prior authorization requirements. Some plans cover assessment under different codes (psychological evaluation, developmental assessment) even if they exclude "autism assessment" specifically.

Payment plan options may be available through private providers. Many understanding providers offer payment plans or sliding scale fees for those with financial constraints. Don't hesitate to discuss your financial situation—many providers want to help and may offer options you didn't know existed.

Health Savings Account (HSA) or Flexible Spending Account (FSA) funds can often be used for autism assessment if you have access to these accounts. Check with your account administrator about eligible expenses.

Grant and scholarship programs occasionally offer funding for autism assessment, particularly through autism organizations or research institutions. While these opportunities are limited, they're worth researching if cost is a significant barrier.

Handling Inconclusive or Incorrect Diagnoses

Not every assessment journey ends with a clear autism diagnosis, and sometimes initial results don't feel accurate. Understanding your options helps you move forward constructively.

Inconclusive results occur when your presentation doesn't clearly meet diagnostic criteria but shows significant autistic traits. This outcome doesn't mean your experiences aren't valid—it might reflect assessment limitations or complex presentations that don't fit neatly into diagnostic categories.

If you receive inconclusive results but still feel autism explains your experiences, consider seeking a second opinion from a provider with more experience in female autism presentations. Dr. Julia Rucklidge's research supports the value of multiple perspectives in complex cases (21).

Incorrect diagnoses sometimes occur when providers miss autism or attribute autistic traits to other conditions. If your diagnosis doesn't feel accurate or doesn't lead to helpful interventions, trust your instincts about seeking additional evaluation.

When pursuing a second opinion, choose a provider with different training or approach from your first assessor. Bring detailed documentation of your experiences and any concerns about the initial assessment.

Self-advocacy strategies become important when navigating assessment challenges. Prepare thoroughly, bring supporting documentation, and don't hesitate to correct misconceptions during the assessment process. Your lived experience matters, and qualified providers should listen to and validate your concerns.

Alternative pathways exist if formal diagnosis remains elusive. Some women find that understanding their autistic traits through self-identification provides sufficient insight for personal growth and self-advocacy, even without formal diagnosis. This approach is valid and increasingly recognized in autism communities (22).

Key Insights Moving Forward

The diagnostic journey represents just one step in understanding yourself as an autistic woman. Whether you receive a formal diagnosis or not, the knowledge you've gained about autism and yourself remains valuable for moving forward authentically.

Professional diagnosis can open doors to accommodations, services, and validation, but it doesn't define your worth or determine your future. Many women find that the assessment process itself—the opportunity to discuss their experiences with a knowledgeable provider—offers clarity and validation regardless of the final diagnosis.

Your journey continues beyond assessment, incorporating this new understanding into your daily life, relationships, and self-care practices. The next phase involves processing your diagnosis emotionally and beginning to integrate this knowledge into your identity and life decisions.

Chapter 3: Processing Your Diagnosis

Emotional Integration

Receiving an autism diagnosis in midlife triggers a cascade of emotions that can feel overwhelming and contradictory. You might experience relief at finally having answers alongside grief for the years spent struggling without understanding why. This emotional journey is normal, necessary, and ultimately healing when approached with patience and self-compassion.

Dr. Kieran Rose, an autistic researcher, describes late diagnosis as simultaneously liberating and devastating—liberating because it provides explanations for lifelong challenges, devastating because it highlights years of unnecessary struggle (23). Understanding this emotional complexity helps normalize your experience and guides you through the integration process.

The Grief Cycle of Late Diagnosis

Processing an autism diagnosis follows a grief-like pattern, though not necessarily in linear stages. You're grieving the life you thought you had while celebrating the understanding you've gained. This paradox creates emotional turbulence that requires time and support to navigate.

Relief often arrives first. Finally, your experiences make sense. The exhaustion after social events, the sensory overwhelm in crowded spaces, the intense interests that others found peculiar—everything has an explanation. Maria, diagnosed at 41, described this relief as "puzzle pieces clicking into place after decades of confusion."

This relief can be profound and immediate. You're not broken, difficult, or antisocial. Your brain works differently, and now you understand how. Many women describe feeling validated for the first time in their lives, as if someone finally sees and understands their internal experience.

Anger typically follows close behind. Anger at healthcare providers who missed the signs, teachers who labeled you as "difficult," family members who told you to "try harder," and a society that failed to recognize your needs. This anger is justified and healthy—it represents your emotional system processing years of invalidation and misunderstanding.

Jennifer, diagnosed at 38, struggled with intense anger toward her childhood school system. "They knew I was different but focused on making me conform rather than understanding why I struggled. I lost years of potential support because no one recognized autism in a quiet, compliant girl."

The anger might extend to yourself for masking so effectively that you lost touch with your authentic self. Self-directed anger can be particularly painful because it adds shame to an already complex emotional mix. Remember that masking was a survival strategy, not a character flaw.

Sadness and mourning emerge as you process lost opportunities. You might grieve the friendships that ended because you couldn't navigate unspoken social rules, the careers you didn't pursue because sensory environments felt impossible, or the years spent thinking you were fundamentally flawed.

This mourning process includes grieving the neurotypical life you thought you were supposed to have. The spontaneous social gatherings that drained you, the career paths that didn't align with your sensory needs, the relationships that required constant performance—recognizing these losses is part of accepting your authentic self.

Acceptance develops gradually as you integrate autism into your identity. This doesn't mean accepting limitations— it means accepting yourself as autistic and recognizing both the challenges and strengths this brings. Acceptance allows you to stop fighting your natural tendencies and start working with them.

Reframing Your Life Story

An autism diagnosis provides a new lens through which to view your entire life history. Events, relationships, and experiences that seemed confusing or painful often make perfect sense when understood through an autistic perspective.

Childhood experiences take on new meaning when reframed through autism understanding. The teacher who said you were "in your own world" wasn't criticizing your character—she was observing your natural autistic state. The birthday parties that overwhelmed you weren't evidence of social anxiety—they reflected sensory overload and social confusion typical of autism.

Lisa, now 45, reexamined her childhood through her autism diagnosis. "I always thought I was a weird kid who couldn't make friends normally. Now I realize I was an autistic kid trying to navigate a neurotypical world without any support or understanding. That reframing changed everything."

Academic and professional struggles often reflect accommodations you needed but never received. Difficulty with group projects might have stemmed from communication differences, not lack of cooperation. Challenges with open-concept offices could reflect sensory sensitivities, not antisocial tendencies.

Understanding these connections helps release self-blame and shame you may have carried for years. You weren't lazy, difficult, or antisocial—you were an undiagnosed autistic person doing your best in environments that didn't match your neurological needs.

Relationship patterns become clearer when viewed through an autism lens. The intense friendships that burned out quickly might reflect autistic communication styles and energy management needs. The romantic relationships that felt like constant performance could indicate masking fatigue and difficulty with neurotypical social expectations (24).

Career choices and changes often align perfectly with autistic traits when reexamined. The jobs you thrived in likely provided structure, clear expectations, and aligned with your interests or strengths. The positions that felt impossible probably involved excessive social demands, sensory challenges, or ambiguous expectations.

Addressing Internalized Ableism and Shame

Years of trying to fit neurotypical expectations often result in internalized ableism—unconscious negative beliefs about autism and disability. Processing these internalized messages is essential for authentic self-acceptance and mental health.

Internalized ableism manifests in thoughts like "I'm not really autistic because I'm successful" or "I should be able to handle this because others can." These messages reflect societal prejudices about autism rather than accurate understanding of autistic experiences.

Challenge these thoughts by examining their origins. Who taught you that needing accommodations means weakness? Where did you learn that stimming or special interests are inappropriate? Often, these messages came from well-meaning people who didn't understand autism, not from objective reality.

Shame around stimming, special interests, and sensory needs requires particular attention. You might have learned to suppress these natural behaviors to avoid judgment or correction. Reclaiming these aspects of yourself is both healing and necessary for authentic living.

Practice self-compassion when addressing internalized ableism. You developed these beliefs as protective mechanisms in a world that didn't understand or accept autistic traits. Changing deeply held beliefs takes time and patience with yourself.

Autism-positive resources can help counter negative messages you've internalized. Books, blogs, and social media accounts by autistic authors provide alternative perspectives on autism that celebrate neurodiversity rather than pathologizing differences (25).

Telling Others vs. Keeping It Private

Deciding who to tell about your autism diagnosis is deeply personal and depends on your circumstances, relationships, and comfort level. There's no right or wrong approach—only what feels authentic and safe for you.

Consider your motivation for disclosure. Are you seeking understanding and support, or do you feel pressured to explain your differences? Disclosure should serve your needs and well-being, not others' curiosity or expectations.

Start with safe people when you decide to share your diagnosis. These might be close friends, family members, or colleagues who've shown understanding about differences and challenges. Test the waters with one or two trusted individuals before broader disclosure.

Prepare for varied reactions when you share your diagnosis. Some people will be supportive and curious to learn more. Others might minimize your experience ("You don't seem autistic") or offer unhelpful advice ("Have you tried...?"). These reactions reflect their knowledge and comfort with autism, not the validity of your diagnosis.

Rachel, diagnosed at 35, developed scripts for different disclosure scenarios. "I had prepared responses for common reactions. When people said I didn't 'look autistic,' I explained that autism in women often looks different than stereotypes suggest. It helped me feel more confident sharing my diagnosis."

Workplace disclosure requires particular consideration. Research your company's disability policies and consider whether disclosure might lead to beneficial accommodations or potential discrimination. You're not required to disclose your autism to employers, but doing so can open doors to support and understanding.

Family disclosure can be especially complex, particularly if family members struggle to understand autism or feel defensive about missed signs during your childhood.

Approach these conversations with patience and prepare for the possibility that some family members may need time to process and accept your diagnosis.

Finding Your Autistic Community

Connecting with other autistic adults, particularly women with similar experiences, provides validation, support, and practical strategies for navigating life authentically. This community connection often becomes a cornerstone of post-diagnosis healing and growth.

Online communities offer accessibility and anonymity that can feel safer when you're newly diagnosed. Facebook groups, Twitter communities, and forums specifically for autistic women provide spaces to ask questions, share experiences, and learn from others who understand your journey.

Look for communities that emphasize neurodiversity and autism acceptance rather than cure-focused or deficit-based perspectives. These positive communities celebrate autistic traits while acknowledging challenges, creating environments that support authentic self-expression.

Local support groups may exist in your area through autism organizations, universities, or mental health centers. While these groups might be smaller, they offer face-to-face connection and potential friendships with people who share similar experiences.

Professional networks for autistic adults exist in many fields and can provide career support alongside social connection. These groups understand the unique challenges autistic professionals face and often share strategies for workplace success.

Mentorship relationships with other autistic women can provide invaluable guidance as you navigate post-diagnosis life. Connecting with someone who's further along in their autism journey can offer perspective, hope, and practical advice for challenges you're facing.

Be patient with community connections. Building relationships takes time, and autistic social communication styles might differ from neurotypical relationship patterns. Focus on authentic connections rather than trying to build a large social network.

Moving from "What's Wrong with Me" to "How Does My Brain Work"

The most significant shift in processing your diagnosis involves changing your fundamental perspective from deficit-based thinking to difference-based understanding. This reframe transforms autism from a disorder to overcome into a neurological variation to understand and accommodate.

Deficit-based thinking focuses on what autism prevents you from doing or how it creates challenges. This perspective, while acknowledging real difficulties, can lead to shame, self-criticism, and endless attempts to "fix" yourself. It's the voice that says "I should be able to handle this" or "Normal people don't struggle with this."

Difference-based thinking recognizes autism as a different way of processing and experiencing the world, with both strengths and challenges. This perspective asks "How can I work with my brain rather than against it?" and "What accommodations would help me thrive?"

Sarah, diagnosed at 34, described this shift: "Instead of asking why I couldn't handle loud restaurants, I started asking what environments help me feel comfortable and connected. That question led to much better solutions and less self-criticism."

Practical applications of this reframe affect daily decisions and long-term planning. Instead of forcing yourself into neurotypical social patterns, you might seek out communities and activities that align with your communication style and interests. Rather than pushing through sensory discomfort, you might prioritize environments that support your sensory needs.

Strength identification becomes possible when you stop viewing autistic traits as deficits. Your attention to detail might be a professional asset. Your pattern recognition skills could guide important decisions. Your direct communication style might create more authentic relationships.

This reframe doesn't minimize real challenges or suggest that positive thinking solves everything. Autism can create significant difficulties in a world designed for neurotypical brains. However, understanding these challenges as mismatches between your needs and environmental demands—rather than personal failings—opens possibilities for effective solutions and accommodations.

Moving Forward with Integration

Processing your autism diagnosis is an ongoing journey rather than a destination. You'll continue discovering new aspects of how autism affects your life, and your understanding will deepen over time. This gradual integration is normal and healthy.

Self-compassion remains essential throughout this process. You're learning about yourself in ways that most people never have to consider. Be patient with yourself as you explore what autism means for your relationships, career, and daily life.

Professional support can be invaluable during the integration process. Therapists who understand autism in women can help you process complex emotions, develop coping strategies, and work through relationship challenges that arise from your new understanding.

The next phase of your journey involves practical applications of your autism knowledge—learning how to unmask safely, accommodate your sensory needs, and build authentic relationships that honor your autistic self. Your diagnosis provides the foundation for this work, but the real transformation happens as you begin living authentically as an autistic woman.

Essential Insights for Your Journey

Understanding and processing your autism diagnosis represents a profound shift in self-knowledge that ripples through every aspect of your life. This process takes time, patience, and often professional support, but it ultimately leads to greater self-acceptance and authentic living.

The emotional complexity you're experiencing is not only normal but necessary for healthy integration of your diagnosis into your identity. Allow yourself to feel the full range of emotions without judgment, knowing that each feeling serves a purpose in your healing and growth process.

Your autism diagnosis doesn't change who you are—it provides language and understanding for who you've always been. This knowledge empowers you to make choices that align with your neurological needs rather than fighting against them, opening possibilities for a more authentic and satisfying life.

Key Takeaways:

- Late autism diagnosis triggers complex emotions including relief, anger, grief, and ultimately acceptance

- Reframing your life story through an autism lens reduces self-blame and increases self-understanding

- Internalized ableism requires active work to overcome and replace with autism-positive perspectives

- Disclosure decisions should prioritize your safety, well-being, and authentic relationships over others' expectations

- Connecting with autistic communities provides validation, support, and practical strategies for thriving

- Shifting from deficit-based to difference-based thinking transforms autism from a problem to solve into a neurotype to understand and accommodate

Chapter 4: Unmasking Safely

- Authentic Self-Expression

The mask you've worn for years feels like a second skin—so familiar that removing it seems impossible, even dangerous. Yet beneath this carefully constructed facade lies your authentic self, waiting for permission to exist without apology or explanation. Learning to unmask safely requires both courage and strategy, balancing authenticity with practical considerations about where, when, and how to let your real self emerge.

For decades, you've perfected the art of appearing neurotypical. You've studied social scripts, practiced facial expressions, and suppressed natural behaviors that felt too different or too much. This performance has served you well in many ways—helping you navigate school, work, and relationships that might otherwise have been impossible. But masking comes at a cost that becomes increasingly difficult to ignore as you understand your autism more clearly.

Understanding Masking and Its Origins

Masking develops as an adaptive response to social pressure, rejection, or the simple observation that your natural ways of being don't match what others expect. Most autistic girls begin masking before they even understand what they're doing—they just know that certain behaviors lead to acceptance while others result in correction or exclusion (26).

The process often starts innocuously. A teacher tells you to sit still, so you learn to suppress your need to move.

Classmates laugh at your intense interest in butterflies, so you learn to hide your enthusiasm. Family members correct your "weird" way of talking, so you study how others speak and adopt their patterns. Each interaction teaches you that your authentic self isn't quite right.

Sarah's masking journey began in elementary school when her teacher repeatedly told her to "use her inside voice." Sarah naturally spoke with passion and volume about topics she loved, but this enthusiasm was seen as disruptive. She learned to monitor her voice constantly, speaking so quietly that people often asked her to repeat herself. By middle school, this monitoring had extended to her body language, facial expressions, and even her interests.

Dr. Julia Rood's research identifies three primary masking categories: behavioral masking (suppressing stimming, forcing eye contact), cognitive masking (learning social scripts, mimicking others), and emotional masking (hiding meltdowns, appearing calm when overwhelmed) (27). Most women engage in all three types, creating elaborate systems for appearing neurotypical.

Behavioral masking involves controlling your physical self in ways that feel unnatural. You might force yourself to make eye contact despite the discomfort, suppress the urge to stim when anxious, or sit still during meetings when your body craves movement. These behaviors require constant conscious effort and drain cognitive resources throughout the day.

Cognitive masking requires intense mental energy to decode social situations, plan appropriate responses, and monitor your performance constantly. You develop internal scripts for common social scenarios, study others' facial expressions to mirror them, and calculate the "right" amount of enthusiasm to show about different topics.

Emotional masking involves hiding your authentic emotional responses and displaying what others expect to see. You smile when overwhelmed, appear calm during sensory overload, and suppress meltdowns until you reach privacy. This type of masking can be particularly damaging because it disconnects you from your own emotional experiences.

The Hidden Costs of Constant Performance

Masking isn't just exhausting—it's actively harmful to your physical and mental health. The constant vigilance required to monitor and adjust your behavior creates chronic stress that manifests in various ways throughout your body and mind (28).

Physical costs accumulate over years of suppressing natural movements and maintaining unnatural postures. Forcing yourself to sit still when you need to move creates muscle tension and fatigue. Suppressing stims removes your natural regulation mechanisms, leading to increased anxiety and overwhelm. Many women report chronic pain, headaches, and digestive issues that improve once they begin unmasking.

Mental health impacts include increased rates of anxiety, depression, and eating disorders among autistic women who mask heavily. The constant effort to appear neurotypical while suppressing your authentic self creates internal conflict and disconnection from your own needs and preferences (29). You might lose touch with your own opinions, interests, and even identity.

Autistic burnout represents the ultimate cost of prolonged masking. This state of physical and emotional exhaustion goes beyond typical tiredness—it's a complete depletion of your ability to function at previous levels. Simple tasks become overwhelming, sensory sensitivities increase, and the masking strategies that once felt automatic require enormous effort to maintain (30).

Lisa's burnout experience illustrates this phenomenon clearly. At 35, she was a successful marketing director who prided herself on her ability to "fit in" at work. She attended every happy hour, participated in small talk, and never disclosed her sensory needs. After a particularly demanding project involving multiple presentations and team events, she found herself unable to leave her apartment for three weeks. Basic tasks like grocery shopping felt impossible, and sounds that had never bothered her became unbearable.

The relationship between masking and burnout isn't coincidental—masking depletes the cognitive and emotional resources you need to function effectively. Recognizing this connection helps you understand that unmasking isn't optional for long-term wellbeing; it's necessary for sustainable functioning.

Identifying Your Personal Masking Patterns

Before you can begin unmasking, you need to identify what masking looks like in your specific life. These patterns often feel so automatic that recognizing them requires deliberate attention and reflection.

Social masking strategies might include rehearsing conversations before social events, studying others' body language to copy appropriate responses, or developing scripts for common interactions. You might find yourself agreeing with opinions you don't actually share or expressing enthusiasm for activities that don't interest you.

Professional masking often involves suppressing stims during meetings, forcing yourself to attend social work events, or hiding sensory needs to appear "professional." You might volunteer for projects that overwhelm you to prove your capability or avoid requesting accommodations that would actually help you perform better.

Family masking can be particularly complex because family members knew you before you developed sophisticated masking strategies. You might find yourself reverting to childhood patterns or working extra hard to appear "normal" during family gatherings. Some women mask so effectively that family members refuse to believe their autism diagnosis.

Create a masking inventory by tracking your behaviors across different environments. Notice situations where you feel like you're performing versus times when you feel authentic. Pay attention to activities that drain your energy disproportionately and relationships that require constant effort to maintain.

Ask yourself these reflection questions:

- In which situations do I feel most like myself?

- What behaviors do I suppress or monitor constantly?

- Which relationships require the most effort to maintain?

- What activities leave me feeling drained despite seeming "easy" to others?

- How do I act differently in various social contexts?

Janet's masking assessment revealed surprising patterns. She discovered that she spoke with a higher pitch at work than at home, suppressed her natural tendency to organize things by color and texture, and pretended to enjoy background music that actually caused her significant distress. These realizations helped her identify specific areas where she could begin experimenting with greater authenticity.

Creating Safe Spaces for Authenticity

Unmasking requires safe environments where you can experiment with authentic self-expression without facing negative consequences. These spaces allow you to reconnect with your natural behaviors and preferences while building confidence for gradual expansion into other areas of your life.

Home as your primary sanctuary should accommodate your sensory needs, interests, and natural behaviors without compromise. This might mean adjusting lighting to reduce harsh glare, organizing spaces according to your preferences, or creating quiet zones where you can retreat when overwhelmed. Your home should be the place where masking becomes unnecessary.

Trusted relationships provide interpersonal safety for authentic expression. These might include close friends who accept your stims, family members who understand your communication style, or romantic partners who support your sensory needs. Start by being honest about your autism diagnosis and specific traits with people who've shown understanding and acceptance.

36

Online communities offer anonymity and connection with others who share similar experiences. Autism-focused social media groups, forums, and virtual support meetings allow you to express yourself authentically without worrying about face-to-face social expectations. Many women find their first experiences of unmasked interaction happen in these digital spaces.

Professional support from autism-informed therapists provides structured environments for exploring authentic self-expression. These professionals understand masking patterns and can guide you through the unmasking process while addressing any anxiety or identity confusion that arises.

Nature and solitary activities often provide natural unmasking opportunities. Many autistic women find that time alone in natural settings allows their authentic self to emerge without social pressure. This might mean stimming freely during solo walks, engaging with special interests without time constraints, or simply existing without monitoring your behavior.

Gradual Unmasking Strategies

Successful unmasking happens gradually, with careful attention to your comfort level and the safety of different environments. Rushing this process can lead to overwhelming exposure or negative reactions that make you retreat back into heavy masking.

Start with low-stakes environments where negative reactions have minimal consequences. This might mean stimming during phone calls when others can't see you, expressing your authentic opinions in online spaces, or organizing your personal space according to your preferences rather than social expectations.

Practice authentic behaviors in trusted relationships before expanding to professional or casual social contexts. You might share your special interests with close friends, explain your sensory needs to family members, or discuss your autism diagnosis with your romantic partner. These experiences build confidence and help you develop language for explaining your needs.

Implement sensory accommodations gradually in various environments. Start with small changes like wearing noise-canceling headphones in public, choosing restaurants based on lighting and sound levels, or requesting specific seating arrangements during meetings. These accommodations support your authentic functioning while demonstrating to yourself and others that your needs matter.

Experiment with communication styles that feel more natural to you. This might mean asking direct questions instead of engaging in small talk, sharing enthusiasm about your interests without apologizing, or requesting clarification when social expectations aren't clear. Practice these communication patterns in safe relationships first.

Honor your energy patterns by scheduling activities according to your actual capacity rather than external expectations. This might mean declining social invitations when you're overwhelmed, taking breaks during long meetings, or establishing routines that support your functioning rather than fighting against your natural rhythms.

Rebecca's gradual approach provides a practical example. She started by allowing herself to stim with a small fidget toy during work meetings, keeping it hidden under the table. After several weeks without negative reactions, she began stimming more openly during phone calls. Eventually, she explained to her team that the movement helped her focus, and they accommodated her need without question.

Establishing Healthy Boundaries

Learning to unmask successfully requires clear boundaries about when masking is necessary versus optional. This discernment helps you conserve energy for situations that truly require performance while allowing authentic expression whenever possible.

Safety-based masking may be necessary in situations where authentic autistic behavior could lead to discrimination, job loss, or social rejection with serious consequences. These decisions should be pragmatic rather than shame-based, recognizing that strategic masking can be a survival tool when used consciously.

Professional environments often require some level of masking, but you can usually find opportunities for greater authenticity. This might mean requesting accommodations for sensory needs, finding ways to incorporate your interests into your work, or building relationships with colleagues who appreciate direct communication.

Social situations vary widely in their safety for authentic expression. Family gatherings might require different strategies than casual friendships or romantic relationships. Learning to assess each social context helps you make conscious choices about your level of authenticity rather than defaulting to heavy masking in all situations.

Energy management becomes critical when establishing masking boundaries. High-masking situations should be balanced with opportunities for authentic expression and recovery. This might mean scheduling downtime after challenging social events or ensuring you have spaces for unmasking throughout your day.

Create clear criteria for assessing masking decisions:

1. What are the potential consequences of authentic behavior in this situation?

2. How much energy do I have available for masking right now?

3. What accommodations could reduce my need to mask here?

4. Is this a relationship or environment worth the energy investment?

5. How can I recover after high-masking situations?

Managing Others' Reactions

As you begin expressing yourself more authentically, you'll encounter various reactions from people who knew you primarily through your masked presentation. Preparing for these responses helps you maintain confidence in your unmasking journey.

Positive reactions often come from people who appreciate authenticity and may have sensed that you were holding back aspects of yourself. These individuals might express relief that you're "finally being yourself" or curiosity about learning more about autism. These reactions validate your decision to unmask and often lead to deeper, more satisfying relationships.

Confused reactions typically arise when people notice changes in your behavior but don't understand the context. Family members might comment that you seem different, colleagues might ask about your new fidget toys, or friends might wonder why you're suddenly expressing strong opinions about topics you previously avoided. Clear, simple explanations often resolve this confusion.

Negative reactions unfortunately occur sometimes, particularly from people who benefited from your people-pleasing masked behaviors or who hold prejudiced views about autism. These reactions might include criticism of your "new" behaviors, attempts to shame you back into masking, or even relationship ending because of your authenticity.

Prepare standard responses for common situations:

- "I'm learning to accommodate my sensory needs better."

- "I've always been autistic; I'm just masking less now."

- "This helps me focus and be more present."

- "I'm working on being more authentic in my relationships."

Maria's experience with family reactions illustrates both challenges and successes. When she began stimming openly during family dinners, her mother initially criticized the behavior as "strange" and "attention-seeking." However, after Maria explained that the movement helped her stay calm and present during social gatherings, her mother not only accepted it but began advocating for Maria's needs with other family members.

Set clear expectations with important people in your life about your unmasking process. Explain that you're not becoming a different person—you're allowing your authentic self to be visible. Some relationships may change as a result, but those that survive will be stronger and more genuine.

Building Authentic Relationships

Unmasking creates opportunities for deeper, more satisfying relationships based on genuine connection rather than performance. This process requires courage to be vulnerable and wisdom to choose relationships that appreciate your authentic self.

Authentic communication involves expressing your genuine thoughts, feelings, and needs rather than saying what you think others want to hear. This might mean sharing your enthusiasm about special interests, asking for clarification when social cues aren't clear, or expressing disagreement when you have different opinions.

Mutual accommodation characterizes healthy relationships with autistic individuals. You accommodate others' social and emotional needs while they accommodate your sensory and communication preferences. This reciprocal adjustment creates relationships that work for everyone involved rather than requiring one person to constantly adapt.

Quality over quantity becomes the guiding principle for authentic relationships. You might find that unmasking leads to fewer but more meaningful connections. The energy you previously spent maintaining superficial relationships becomes available for nurturing deep, genuine bonds with people who appreciate your authentic self.

Clear expectations help both you and others navigate authentic relationships successfully. This might mean explaining your communication style, discussing your sensory needs, or establishing boundaries around social energy and time. These conversations prevent misunderstandings and create frameworks for mutual support.

Looking Ahead with Authenticity

Unmasking represents a lifelong process rather than a destination. Your comfort with authentic expression will continue growing as you gain experience and confidence. Some situations may always require strategic masking, and that's acceptable—the goal is conscious choice rather than automatic performance.

The energy you reclaim through reduced masking becomes available for pursuing interests, building relationships, and engaging in activities that truly fulfill you. This authenticity often leads to improved mental health, better relationships, and a stronger sense of identity and self-worth.

Your unmasking journey contributes to broader autism acceptance by demonstrating that autistic women can be successful, valuable community members while expressing their authentic selves. Each time you stim openly, share your interests enthusiastically, or request accommodations confidently, you help expand others' understanding of what autism looks like.

Reflecting on Authentic Living

The path to authentic self-expression requires both courage and patience. You're undoing years of learned behavior while building new patterns that honor your autistic neurology. This process isn't always linear—you may find yourself masking more heavily during stressful periods or in new environments, and that's perfectly normal.

Your authentic self has always existed beneath the mask. Unmasking doesn't create a new identity—it reveals who you've always been. This distinction is important because it validates your experiences throughout your life, even during periods of heavy masking.

The relationships and environments that support your authentic expression are worth cultivating and protecting. These spaces become foundations for a life that works with your brain rather than against it, creating sustainable patterns for long-term wellbeing and success.

Chapter 5: Sensory Liberation

- Understanding Your Sensory World

Your sensory system processes information differently than neurotypical brains, creating a unique experience of the world that can be both challenging and extraordinarily rich. What others dismiss as "just background noise" might overwhelm your nervous system, while textures that comfort you might feel strange or unpleasant to them. Understanding your sensory profile transforms these differences from mysterious symptoms into predictable patterns you can accommodate and even celebrate.

Traditional medical models focus on sensory issues as problems to fix rather than differences to understand and support. This approach often leaves autistic women feeling broken rather than different. Recent research reveals that sensory differences in autism aren't deficits—they're alternative ways of processing environmental information that require accommodation rather than elimination (31).

The Eight Sensory Systems

Your nervous system processes information through eight distinct sensory channels, not the five traditionally taught in school. Understanding all eight systems helps you identify your specific patterns and develop effective accommodation strategies.

Visual processing affects how you interpret and respond to light, color, movement, and spatial relationships. You might be oversensitive to fluorescent lighting, fascinated by certain patterns, or struggle with depth perception in crowded spaces. Some autistic women find bright lights physically painful, while others seek out specific visual stimulation for regulation.

Auditory processing influences your response to sounds, volume levels, and acoustic environments. Background conversations might feel overwhelming even when others don't notice them, or specific sounds might cause physical discomfort. Conversely, you might find certain sounds incredibly soothing or use specific music for emotional regulation.

Tactile processing governs your response to touch, texture, temperature, and pressure. Clothing tags might feel like constant irritation, while others find deep pressure incredibly calming. Many autistic women have specific fabric preferences or need particular bedding textures for comfortable sleep.

Olfactory and gustatory processing affect smell and taste sensitivities that can significantly impact daily life. Strong scents might trigger headaches or nausea, while specific flavors provide comfort or regulation. Food aversions often relate to texture, temperature, or smell rather than actual taste preferences.

Proprioceptive processing involves body awareness and spatial positioning. You might bump into things frequently, have difficulty gauging force when writing or hugging, or crave activities that provide strong proprioceptive input like heavy lifting or tight hugs. This system often functions differently in autistic individuals.

Vestibular processing affects balance, coordination, and spatial orientation. You might love or hate spinning activities, feel anxious on elevators, or use movement for self-regulation. Changes in head position might affect your comfort level more than others experience.

Interoceptive processing involves awareness of internal body signals like hunger, thirst, fatigue, or bathroom needs. Many autistic women struggle to identify these signals reliably, leading to irregular eating, dehydration, or other health challenges. This system also affects emotional awareness and regulation.

Identifying Your Sensory Profile

Each person has a unique combination of sensory preferences, sensitivities, and seeking behaviors. Identifying your specific patterns helps you understand your reactions and develop personalized accommodation strategies.

Sensory seeking behaviors occur when your nervous system craves certain types of input for regulation or enjoyment. You might touch soft fabrics repeatedly, listen to specific music for hours, or crave spicy foods. These behaviors often serve important regulatory functions even if others find them unusual.

Sensory avoiding behaviors develop when certain inputs feel overwhelming, painful, or distressing. You might cover your ears in restaurants, avoid certain clothing textures, or feel nauseated by specific smells. These reactions are valid neurological responses, not character flaws or overreactions.

Mixed patterns are common, where you seek certain sensory experiences while avoiding others within the same system. You might love soft textures but hate rough ones, enjoy classical music but find rock concerts unbearable, or crave movement but dislike unexpected motion.

Jennifer's sensory assessment revealed complex patterns that explained years of mysterious reactions. She discovered that she sought proprioceptive input through heavy blankets and tight clothing but avoided light touch from others. Auditorily, she found background conversations overwhelming but used specific nature sounds for concentration. Understanding these patterns helped her modify her environment for better functioning.

Track your sensory responses systematically by noting reactions across different environments and times of day. Pay attention to:

- Which environments feel comfortable versus overwhelming

- What sensory experiences you naturally seek out

- Which situations you instinctively avoid

- How sensory experiences affect your mood and energy

- What sensory strategies help you feel regulated

Sensory journals can reveal patterns that aren't immediately obvious. Note your comfort levels in different environments, energy changes after sensory experiences, and any physical reactions to specific inputs. These patterns often become clear over time even if daily experiences feel unpredictable.

Creating Sensory-Friendly Environments

Your environment significantly affects your ability to function, regulate emotions, and engage in daily activities. Modifying spaces to support your sensory needs isn't indulgent—it's necessary for optimal functioning and wellbeing.

Home modifications should prioritize your comfort and regulation needs. This might involve changing lighting to reduce harsh glare, using specific textures for furniture and bedding, controlling sound levels, or organizing spaces to reduce visual clutter. Your home should be a sensory sanctuary where you can retreat and recharge.

Lighting adjustments can dramatically improve comfort and functioning. Replace fluorescent bulbs with LED or incandescent alternatives, use dimmer switches to control brightness, add lamps for softer lighting options, or install blackout curtains for darker environments. Many autistic women find that lighting changes alone significantly reduce daily stress.

Sound management helps create acoustic environments that support rather than overwhelm you. Use noise-canceling headphones or earplugs, add sound-absorbing materials like carpets or curtains, create quiet zones for retreat, or use white noise machines to mask unpredictable sounds. Some women find that controlling their acoustic environment improves focus and reduces anxiety dramatically.

Texture considerations extend beyond clothing to furniture, bedding, and household items. Choose fabrics that feel comfortable against your skin, select furniture based on tactile preferences, use specific bedding for better sleep, or add texture elements that provide sensory comfort. These modifications often improve daily comfort significantly.

Workplace accommodations might include adjusting your workspace lighting, using noise-canceling headphones, requesting specific seating arrangements, or modifying dress code requirements. Many employers are willing to make reasonable accommodations once they understand how sensory modifications improve productivity and comfort.

Susan's office transformation illustrates effective workplace modifications. She replaced the overhead fluorescent lighting with a desk lamp, added a small carpet under her desk for texture variety, used noise-canceling headphones during focused work, and requested permission to work from a quieter location during particularly demanding projects. These changes improved her productivity and reduced end-of-day exhaustion significantly.

Sensory Tools and Accommodations

Specific tools and strategies can help you manage sensory challenges and enhance comfortable sensory experiences. These accommodations should be viewed as necessary supports rather than optional preferences.

Auditory tools help manage sound-related challenges and provide beneficial auditory input. Noise-canceling headphones reduce overwhelming background noise, earplugs filter harsh sounds while maintaining speech clarity, white noise apps mask unpredictable sounds, or specific music playlists provide regulation and comfort.

Tactile tools offer ways to seek beneficial touch input or avoid uncomfortable sensations. Fidget toys provide discrete tactile stimulation, weighted blankets offer proprioceptive comfort, specific fabric choices reduce clothing-related distress, or textured objects provide sensory grounding during overwhelming situations.

Visual accommodations help manage light sensitivity and visual overwhelm. Sunglasses reduce harsh lighting indoors and outdoors, computer screen filters minimize eye strain, specific color filters improve visual comfort, or room modifications reduce visual clutter and distraction.

Proprioceptive supports provide the deep pressure and body awareness that many autistic individuals crave. Exercise equipment offers intense proprioceptive input, compression clothing provides constant gentle pressure, yoga or stretching provides body awareness, or specific movement activities help with regulation.

Olfactory management helps you navigate scent-related challenges while using beneficial smells for regulation. Unscented products reduce overwhelming fragrances, essential oils provide calming or alerting scents, air purifiers reduce environmental odors, or specific scents serve as emotional regulation tools.

Temperature regulation tools help manage thermal sensitivities that affect comfort and functioning. Layered clothing allows quick adjustments, heating pads or cooling items provide comfort, fans or heaters modify environmental temperature, or specific fabrics help maintain comfortable body temperature.

Managing Sensory Overload

Sensory overload occurs when your nervous system receives more input than it can process effectively, leading to overwhelm, shutdown, or meltdown. Understanding your overload patterns helps you identify triggers and develop effective response strategies.

Early warning signs often appear before full overload occurs, giving you opportunities for intervention. These might include increased irritability, difficulty concentrating, physical tension, stronger reactions to normally tolerable stimuli, or unusual fatigue. Learning to recognize these signals allows for proactive management.

Immediate response strategies help manage overload when it occurs. Remove yourself from overwhelming environments when possible, use sensory tools for regulation, practice deep breathing or other calming techniques, engage in familiar self-soothing behaviors, or communicate your needs to others present.

Prevention strategies reduce the likelihood and intensity of sensory overload. Plan breaks during challenging activities, modify environments proactively, use sensory tools preemptively, limit exposure to known triggers, or schedule recovery time after high-sensory situations.

Recovery protocols help you return to baseline functioning after overload episodes. Rest in low-stimulation environments, engage in preferred sensory activities, use familiar comfort items, practice gentle movement or stretching, or allow extra time for emotional and physical recovery.

Amy's overload management demonstrates effective strategy implementation. She learned that crowded restaurants triggered overload within 20 minutes, so she began requesting specific seating areas, using noise-canceling headphones during peak times, taking bathroom breaks for sensory relief, and planning quieter activities after restaurant visits. These modifications allowed her to maintain social connections while protecting her sensory wellbeing.

Sensory Considerations for Daily Life

Integrating sensory awareness into daily decisions transforms routine activities from potential challenges into opportunities for wellbeing and comfort. This approach requires initial planning but becomes automatic with practice.

Clothing choices significantly affect daily comfort and functioning. Select fabrics based on tactile preferences, choose fit that provides comfortable pressure levels, remove or modify irritating elements like tags or seams, or maintain backup clothing options for unexpected sensory challenges. Many women find that addressing clothing sensitivities alone improves their daily mood and energy.

Food considerations extend beyond nutrition to include texture, temperature, smell, and visual presentation. Honor texture preferences without guilt, prepare foods in ways that increase palatability, maintain safe food options for challenging days, or explore new foods gradually to expand preferences safely.

Activity planning should account for sensory demands and recovery needs. Choose restaurants based on acoustic levels, plan outdoor activities considering weather sensitivities, balance high-stimulation events with quiet recovery time, or modify traditional activities to increase sensory comfort.

Transportation considerations help you manage travel-related sensory challenges. Choose seats that minimize unwanted sensory input, bring tools for managing motion sensitivity, plan routes that avoid overwhelming environments, or schedule extra time for sensory adjustment after travel.

Social event modifications allow you to participate in important gatherings while protecting your sensory wellbeing. Arrive early to adjust to environments gradually, identify quiet spaces for breaks, communicate sensory needs to hosts, or plan departure strategies if overload occurs.

Teaching Others About Your Sensory Needs

Helping family members, friends, and colleagues understand your sensory differences creates opportunities for support and accommodation while reducing misunderstandings about your reactions and preferences.

Educational conversations help others understand that sensory differences are neurological variations rather than personal preferences or behavioral choices. Explain how sensory processing affects daily functioning, provide specific examples of your experiences, share resources about sensory differences in autism, or demonstrate how accommodations help you function better.

Specific requests are more effective than general explanations when seeking accommodations. Ask for specific lighting adjustments rather than mentioning light sensitivity generally, request particular seating arrangements instead of discussing crowd aversion broadly, or explain exact sound levels that work versus those that overwhelm.

Family education often requires ongoing conversations as understanding develops gradually. Share information about sensory processing differences, explain how accommodations help the whole family function better, involve family members in identifying environmental modifications, or model sensory self-advocacy for children who might benefit from similar strategies.

Workplace communication should focus on how sensory accommodations improve productivity and job performance. Frame requests in terms of work effectiveness, provide specific accommodation suggestions, offer to trial modifications before permanent implementation, or connect accommodations to business benefits like increased focus and reduced sick days.

Rebecca's family approach shows effective education strategies. She created a simple handout explaining her sensory needs, organized a family meeting to discuss household accommodations, invited family members to experience sensory tools themselves, and celebrated successful accommodations with appreciation and positive reinforcement. This approach led to family-wide support and proactive accommodation offers.

Embracing Sensory Strengths

While sensory differences create challenges, they also provide unique abilities and experiences that can be sources of joy, creativity, and professional advantage. Recognizing and cultivating these strengths balances the focus on accommodation with celebration of neurodiversity.

Enhanced sensory awareness often allows you to notice details that others miss, appreciate subtle environmental changes, identify quality differences in products or experiences, or provide valuable feedback about sensory aspects of environments and products.

Sensory-based skills might include exceptional ability to detect sound differences for music or quality control, visual pattern recognition for design or analysis work, texture discrimination for craft or manufacturing applications, or olfactory sensitivity for cooking or fragrance-related fields.

Aesthetic appreciation can be enhanced by sensory differences, leading to rich experiences with art, music, nature, or other sensory-rich environments. Your sensory profile might allow you to appreciate aspects of beauty that others cannot access or experience.

Professional applications of sensory strengths include careers that utilize your specific sensory abilities, volunteer opportunities that benefit from sensory awareness, creative pursuits that incorporate sensory preferences, or consultation roles helping others understand sensory considerations.

Personal enrichment through sensory experiences can provide deep satisfaction and regulation. This might include specific music that creates profound emotional responses, textures that provide comfort and calm, visual experiences that inspire creativity, or movement activities that enhance wellbeing.

Practical Wisdom for Sensory Success

Understanding your sensory world requires ongoing attention and adjustment as your needs change with circumstances, age, and environmental factors. This awareness becomes a valuable life skill that improves decision-making and self-advocacy across all areas of your life.

Your sensory needs are valid regardless of how they compare to others' experiences. What feels overwhelming to you deserves accommodation even if others find the same stimulus comfortable or enjoyable. Trusting your sensory experiences and advocating for your needs improves both immediate comfort and long-term health outcomes.

Sensory accommodations often benefit others even if they don't share your specific sensitivities. Reducing background noise, improving lighting, or choosing comfortable furniture creates better environments for many people, making your advocacy efforts valuable for entire communities.

The investment in understanding and accommodating your sensory needs pays dividends in improved functioning, better relationships, and enhanced quality of life. These modifications aren't luxuries—they're necessary supports that allow you to engage fully in life while honoring your neurological differences.

Chapter 6: Executive Function Realities

- Practical Life Management

Executive function challenges in autism aren't character flaws or signs of laziness—they're neurological differences that affect how your brain organizes, plans, and executes daily tasks. Understanding these differences allows you to develop systems that work with your brain rather than against it, transforming daily chaos into manageable routines that support your goals and wellbeing.

Traditional productivity advice assumes neurotypical executive function patterns, often leading autistic women to feel inadequate when these strategies fail. The secret lies not in forcing yourself to think differently, but in creating external structures that support your unique cognitive patterns while honoring your strengths and limitations (32).

Understanding Executive Function Differences

Executive function encompasses multiple cognitive processes that work together to help you plan, organize, remember, and complete tasks. In autism, these processes often work differently than in neurotypical brains, creating specific patterns of strengths and challenges that require tailored approaches.

Working memory differences affect your ability to hold multiple pieces of information while completing tasks. You might excel at deep focus on single topics but struggle to remember multi-step instructions or maintain awareness of multiple projects simultaneously. This isn't a memory problem—it's a difference in how your brain processes and prioritizes information.

Task initiation challenges can make starting projects feel impossible even when you understand exactly what needs to be done. This difficulty often intensifies with tasks that lack clear structure, have ambiguous requirements, or involve multiple steps. The "just start" advice that works for neurotypical people often feels meaningless when your brain needs more specific activation strategies.

Time processing differences might affect your perception of duration, ability to estimate task completion times, or awareness of schedules and deadlines. You might become so absorbed in interesting activities that hours pass unnoticed, or find that boring tasks feel endless even when they take only minutes.

Cognitive flexibility challenges can make adapting to unexpected changes particularly difficult. Your brain might process information sequentially rather than simultaneously, making rapid task-switching feel overwhelming or disorienting. This doesn't indicate rigidity—it reflects how your brain optimally processes complex information.

Maria's executive function pattern illustrates these differences clearly. She could research topics for hours with incredible focus and detail but struggled to transition between different types of work throughout the day. Simple tasks like answering emails felt overwhelming when she was deeply engaged in analytical work. Understanding this pattern helped her restructure her schedule to group similar tasks and build in transition time between different cognitive demands.

Time Management Strategies That Honor Your Brain

Effective time management for autistic women requires strategies that account for focus patterns, energy cycles, and processing differences rather than fighting against them. These approaches often differ significantly from conventional time management advice.

Energy-based scheduling prioritizes your natural energy patterns over external demands whenever possible. Identify times when you feel most alert and focused for demanding cognitive work, recognize periods when routine tasks feel more manageable, and protect high-energy times for your most important activities. This approach maximizes your effectiveness while reducing daily stress.

Transition time becomes a crucial component of realistic scheduling. Build buffer periods between different types of activities, allow extra time for shifting between mental tasks, and create rituals that help your brain transition smoothly between different cognitive demands. Many autistic women find that underestimating transition needs leads to chronic scheduling stress.

Hyperfocus management involves working with rather than against periods of intense concentration. When you enter hyperfocus states, set alarms for basic needs like eating or drinking, prepare your environment with necessary supplies beforehand, and protect these periods from interruption when possible. Rather than viewing hyperfocus as problematic, treat it as a valuable cognitive resource to channel effectively.

Time blocking helps create structure while accommodating your focus patterns. Assign specific time periods for different types of work, group similar tasks together to minimize cognitive switching, and build flexibility into your schedule for unexpected focus shifts. This approach provides structure without the rigidity that can feel suffocating.

Visual time tracking makes abstract time concepts more concrete and manageable. Use analog clocks to see time visually, employ countdown timers for specific tasks, create visual schedules that show daily structure, or use color-coding systems to represent different types of activities. Many autistic women find that making time visible reduces anxiety and improves planning accuracy.

Sarah's time management evolution demonstrates these principles in action. She discovered that her peak cognitive hours occurred between 9 AM and noon, so she protected this time for complex analytical work. She built 15-minute transition periods between different task types, used a visual timer during focused work sessions, and scheduled routine tasks during her naturally lower-energy afternoon periods. This alignment between her schedule and her brain's patterns dramatically improved both productivity and wellbeing.

Organization Systems for the Autistic Mind

Effective organization systems for autistic women often emphasize visual clarity, logical categorization, and consistency rather than the minimalist approaches popular in neurotypical productivity culture. Your organizational needs are valid even if they look different from conventional wisdom.

Visual organization makes information immediately accessible without requiring memory retrieval. Use clear containers so you can see contents, label everything with both words and pictures when helpful, organize items by frequency of use rather than arbitrary categories, or create visual maps of where things belong. Many autistic women find that "out of sight, out of mind" affects their ability to use possessions effectively.

Category-based systems align with the pattern-recognition strengths common in autism. Group similar items together consistently, create logical hierarchies for information storage, use consistent naming conventions across all organizational systems, or develop classification systems that make sense to your specific brain. The key is creating systems that feel intuitive to you rather than conforming to external organizational standards.

Routine-based organization reduces daily decision fatigue while maintaining order. Establish consistent places for frequently used items, create standard procedures for common tasks, develop evening and morning routines that maintain organization automatically, or build organizational maintenance into existing habits. This approach makes organization sustainable rather than requiring constant conscious effort.

External memory systems compensate for working memory differences by storing information outside your brain. Use digital tools for task lists and reminders, create physical notebooks for important information, develop consistent filing systems for documents and resources, or establish standard locations for crucial items like keys and phones.

Jennifer's organizational breakthrough came when she stopped trying to implement minimalist systems that left everything hidden. She switched to clear storage containers throughout her home, created detailed labeling systems for her craft supplies, established consistent locations for items based on use patterns rather than aesthetics, and developed visual checklists for multi-step processes. These changes reduced daily stress and improved her ability to maintain organization consistently.

Managing Transitions and Unexpected Changes

Transitions and unexpected changes can be particularly challenging when your brain processes information sequentially and benefits from predictability. Developing strategies for these situations improves flexibility while honoring your processing needs.

Transition rituals help your brain shift between different activities or mental states. Create specific routines for moving between work and personal time, develop standard procedures for leaving and arriving at locations, use consistent cues to signal activity changes, or establish brief mindfulness practices that facilitate mental transitions. These rituals provide structure during naturally chaotic periods.

Change preparation strategies reduce the stress of unexpected modifications to plans or routines. Maintain backup plans for common disruptions, practice mental flexibility through small controlled changes, develop standard responses to typical unexpected situations, or create comfort kits for managing change-related stress.

Information processing time becomes crucial when dealing with unexpected changes. Allow yourself time to process new information before responding, ask clarifying questions to understand changes fully, request written summaries of complex modifications when possible, or communicate your need for processing time to others involved.

Recovery protocols help you return to baseline functioning after challenging transitions or unexpected changes. Plan downtime after demanding change situations, engage in familiar self-soothing activities, return to established routines as soon as possible, or practice self-compassion when changes feel overwhelming.

Lisa's change management system illustrates effective strategies. When her work schedule changed unexpectedly, she gave herself permission to feel stressed rather than forcing immediate acceptance. She asked for written details about the new schedule, spent time planning how to modify her routines accordingly, identified potential challenges and solutions in advance, and scheduled extra self-care during the transition period. This approach helped her adapt successfully while honoring her processing needs.

Breaking Down Overwhelming Tasks

Large or complex tasks can feel impossible when your brain struggles with task initiation or becomes overwhelmed by multiple components. Learning to deconstruct these tasks into manageable pieces makes them accessible while building confidence for future challenges.

Task analysis involves examining overwhelming projects to identify specific, concrete steps. Break large tasks into smaller components that can be completed in single sessions, identify the actual first step rather than staying in planning mode, recognize which parts require different types of cognitive energy, or determine what resources and information you need for each component.

The "next smallest step" approach focuses on identifying the most minimal possible action you can take toward a goal. This might be opening the relevant document, gathering one piece of needed information, or setting up your workspace for the task. These tiny steps overcome initiation difficulties while building momentum.

External structure creation provides the framework that your brain needs for complex tasks. Use project management tools to track components, create physical workspaces dedicated to specific projects, establish deadlines for individual steps rather than only final deadlines, or develop templates for repeated types of complex tasks.

Energy matching aligns task components with your available cognitive resources. Tackle complex analysis during high-energy periods, save routine components for lower-energy times, recognize which tasks require sustained attention versus those that can be interrupted, or batch similar cognitive demands together.

Progress tracking maintains motivation and provides evidence of advancement when large tasks feel endless. Use visual progress indicators like checklists or progress bars, celebrate completion of individual components, take photos of physical progress when applicable, or maintain logs of time spent and work completed.

Rachel's thesis experience demonstrates these strategies effectively. Her 100-page research project felt impossible until she broke it into specific components: research phase, outline creation, individual chapter drafts, revision cycles, and formatting. She further subdivided each chapter into 2-3 page sections, created a visual progress chart, and celebrated each completed section. This approach transformed an overwhelming project into a series of manageable tasks.

Using Special Interests and Routines as Supports

Your special interests and preference for routines aren't obstacles to productivity—they're powerful tools that can enhance your executive functioning when leveraged effectively. These strengths can provide motivation, structure, and energy for tackling challenging tasks.

Interest-based motivation harnesses your natural enthusiasm to fuel difficult tasks. Connect boring projects to aspects that genuinely interest you, research the background or context of required tasks to find engaging elements, gamify routine activities using themes from your interests, or reward task completion with time spent on preferred activities.

Routine as structure provides the external framework that supports executive functioning. Establish consistent daily routines that include both preferred and necessary activities, create standard procedures for recurring tasks, use familiar patterns to anchor new or challenging activities, or build flexibility into routines rather than making them completely rigid.

Special interest expertise can enhance work performance and provide career direction. Leverage deep knowledge in your interest areas for professional advantage, use pattern recognition skills developed through special interests for problem-solving, apply research skills from exploring interests to work projects, or find career paths that align with your areas of passionate expertise.

Routine-based task initiation overcomes start-up difficulties by embedding challenging tasks within familiar patterns. Begin difficult tasks immediately after established routine activities, create consistent environments and setups for different types of work, use the same tools and materials in predictable ways, or establish reward patterns that follow task completion.

Amanda's integration approach shows these strategies in practice. Her special interest in historical fashion became a motivational tool for her marketing job—she researched the historical context of brand aesthetics, connected design principles to historical periods she loved, and rewarded completing difficult projects with research time on costume history. She also established morning routines that naturally led into work tasks, making task initiation feel automatic rather than effortful.

Technology Tools for Executive Function Support

Digital tools can provide the external structure and reminders that support executive functioning when chosen and configured thoughtfully. The key is finding tools that enhance your existing systems rather than creating additional complexity.

Task management applications help externalize memory and provide visual organization. Choose apps that match your thinking style, use visual elements like colors and categories, set realistic reminder frequencies that don't become overwhelming, or integrate with other tools you already use consistently. The best task management system is the one you'll actually use regularly.

Calendar integration makes time management more concrete and reduces scheduling conflicts. Use visual calendars that show time blocks clearly, color-code different types of activities, set multiple reminders for important events, or integrate calendar systems across devices for consistent access. Many autistic women benefit from seeing their entire schedule visually rather than keeping mental track of commitments.

Automation tools reduce daily decision fatigue by handling routine tasks automatically. Set up automatic bill payments for consistent expenses, use email filters to organize incoming messages, create template responses for common communications, or automate social media posting for business purposes. These tools free cognitive resources for more important decisions.

Focus applications support sustained attention and manage distractions effectively. Use website blockers during focused work time, try ambient sound apps that enhance concentration, employ timer applications that structure work and break periods, or utilize distraction-blocking tools that align with your specific focus challenges.

Note-taking systems externalize information storage and support knowledge management. Choose digital or physical systems based on your preferences, develop consistent formatting for different types of information, create searchable systems for easy information retrieval, or integrate note-taking with task management for seamless workflow.

Michelle's technology integration exemplifies thoughtful tool selection. She used a visual task management app that allowed her to see all projects at once, integrated her calendar with automatic reminders set for optimal timing, employed a note-taking system that connected to her task lists, and used focus apps during her peak concentration hours. This technology stack supported her executive functioning without creating additional management burden.

Building Sustainable Systems

Effective executive function support requires systems that you can maintain consistently over time rather than complex solutions that work temporarily but become overwhelming. Sustainability should be a primary consideration when developing any organizational or time management approach.

Start small and build gradually rather than implementing complete system overhauls that feel overwhelming. Choose one area of executive function to address first, develop simple initial systems that require minimal maintenance, test approaches for several weeks before adding complexity, or modify existing habits rather than creating entirely new routines.

Regular system maintenance keeps organizational approaches functional over time. Schedule weekly reviews of task lists and organizational systems, adjust systems based on what's working and what isn't, simplify approaches that become too complex to maintain, or update tools and categories as your life circumstances change.

Flexibility within structure allows systems to accommodate changes without complete breakdown. Build buffer time into schedules for unexpected demands, create backup plans for common disruptions, allow some categories in organizational systems to be flexible, or develop multiple approaches for different circumstances rather than relying on single solutions.

Energy-aware sustainability acknowledges that your executive functioning capacity varies with stress, health, and life circumstances. Create simplified versions of systems for low-energy periods, identify which system components are essential versus optional, develop emergency protocols for overwhelming periods, or build recovery time into demanding schedules.

Self-compassion in system failure recognizes that all systems occasionally break down and that this doesn't represent personal failure. Expect periodic system maintenance and adjustment, plan for times when you can't maintain usual standards, develop strategies for getting back on track after disruptions, or focus on progress rather than perfection in system implementation.

Practical Wisdom for Executive Function Success

Understanding your executive function patterns provides a foundation for making decisions that support rather than exhaust your cognitive resources. This awareness becomes increasingly valuable as you build systems that truly work for your unique brain.

Your executive function differences are neurological variations, not character flaws or evidence of inadequate effort. The strategies that work for neurotypical individuals may not be effective for you, and that's expected rather than problematic. Finding approaches that align with your cognitive patterns is a skill that improves with practice and self-awareness.

Effective executive function support often looks different from conventional productivity advice. Visual organization might be more important than minimalism, routine might be more valuable than flexibility, and interest-based motivation might be more sustainable than discipline-based approaches. Trust your experience over external expectations about how organization should look.

The investment in understanding and supporting your executive functioning pays significant dividends in reduced stress, improved task completion, and better overall life management. These systems aren't luxuries—they're necessary accommodations that allow you to function effectively while honoring your neurological differences.

Key Insights for Moving Forward:

- Executive function differences in autism require personalized strategies rather than universal productivity solutions

- Energy-based scheduling and visual organization often work better than conventional time management approaches

- Special interests and routines can be powerful tools for motivation and structure when leveraged thoughtfully

- Technology tools should enhance existing systems rather than create additional complexity

- Sustainable systems prioritize consistency over perfection and build in flexibility for life's inevitable changes

- Self-compassion during system breakdowns supports long-term success better than self-criticism

Chapter 7: Marriage and Partnership

- Intimate Relationships Post-Diagnosis

Your autism diagnosis changes everything and nothing about your relationship simultaneously. The person your partner fell in love with hasn't changed—but now you both have a framework for understanding communication patterns, sensory needs, and emotional responses that may have seemed mysterious or challenging before. This new knowledge creates opportunities for deeper connection and more effective partnership, though it also requires honest conversations and mutual adjustments.

Many autistic women worry that their diagnosis will negatively affect their romantic relationships. Research by Dr. Amy Gravino shows that couples who approach autism as a neurological difference to understand rather than a problem to solve often experience improved intimacy and communication (33). The key lies not in changing who you are, but in helping your partner understand how your brain works so you can build accommodation and appreciation into your relationship.

Explaining Your Diagnosis to Your Partner

Sharing your autism diagnosis with your romantic partner represents a significant moment of vulnerability that can deepen your connection or create temporary confusion as you both process this new information. The conversation itself matters less than the ongoing dialogue that follows.

Choose your timing carefully when planning this conversation. Avoid periods of high stress, major life changes, or relationship conflict. Select a time when you both have emotional energy available and won't be interrupted by work, children, or other commitments. This conversation deserves your full attention and shouldn't feel rushed.

Prepare key information to help your partner understand what autism means for you specifically. Avoid overwhelming them with general autism information and focus on how your traits manifest in daily life. Explain your sensory sensitivities, communication preferences, social energy patterns, and specific strengths that autism brings to your relationship.

Address their concerns directly while validating any confusion or worry they might experience. Partners often wonder if they've done something wrong, if the relationship will change dramatically, or if your diagnosis explains past conflicts. Reassure them that you're the same person they've always known, but now you both have better tools for understanding and supporting each other.

Sarah's disclosure conversation illustrates effective approaches. She chose a quiet evening at home, prepared specific examples of how autism affected her daily experiences, and explained that her diagnosis was an explanation rather than an excuse for relationship challenges. She emphasized that understanding her autism would help them work together more effectively rather than changing their fundamental dynamic.

Provide educational resources that help your partner learn about autism in women without making them responsible for becoming experts. Share books, articles, or videos that present autism positively while acknowledging real challenges. Choose resources that focus on strengths and accommodation rather than deficit-based perspectives.

Allow processing time for your partner to absorb this information and formulate questions. They might need days or weeks to fully understand what your diagnosis means for your relationship. Be patient with their learning process while maintaining boundaries around respectful language and attitudes toward autism.

Communication Patterns in Autistic-Neurotypical Relationships

Autism affects communication in specific ways that can either create misunderstanding or become sources of connection when both partners understand these differences. Your direct communication style, need for clarity, and processing patterns are neurological traits that can actually strengthen relationships when accommodated appropriately.

Direct communication styles often characterize autistic communication and can be refreshing in romantic relationships when partners understand this trait. Your tendency to say what you mean, ask for what you need, and express genuine opinions creates opportunities for authentic connection that many neurotypical relationships lack.

However, neurotypical partners might initially interpret direct communication as rudeness or criticism. Help them understand that your straightforward style reflects honesty and trust rather than lack of consideration. You feel safe enough with them to communicate authentically rather than performing social politeness.

Processing time differences affect how you participate in conversations, make decisions, and respond to unexpected situations. You might need longer to formulate responses to complex questions, time to think through decisions that your partner makes quickly, or space to process emotional information before discussing it.

Lisa's communication breakthrough occurred when she explained to her husband that her delayed responses to his questions weren't signs of disinterest—they reflected her careful thought process. Once he understood this pattern, he began asking important questions via text first, giving her processing time before verbal discussions. This accommodation improved both their satisfaction with communication.

Sensory communication factors influence how you prefer to communicate and what environments support effective conversation. Background noise might make listening difficult, certain lighting might affect your ability to focus on facial expressions, or physical proximity might feel overwhelming during serious discussions.

Emotional expression differences might affect how you show and interpret feelings in your relationship. You might express love through actions rather than words, show excitement differently than neurotypical expectations suggest, or need specific reassurance about your partner's emotional state when their cues aren't clear to you.

Create communication agreements that honor both your needs and your partner's preferences. This might include scheduling important conversations during your optimal times, using written communication for complex topics, establishing clear signals for when you need processing time, or developing backup communication methods for challenging situations.

Sensory Considerations in Physical Intimacy

Physical intimacy involves complex sensory experiences that can be intensely pleasurable or overwhelmingly uncomfortable for autistic individuals. Understanding and accommodating your sensory needs creates space for satisfying physical connection while avoiding experiences that cause distress or shutdown.

Touch sensitivity variations affect how you experience physical contact throughout your body and across different times and circumstances. You might crave deep pressure touch but find light stroking uncomfortable, enjoy specific textures against your skin while avoiding others, or have particular areas of your body that feel especially sensitive or pleasurable.

Environmental sensory factors significantly influence your comfort with physical intimacy. Lighting levels might affect your ability to relax and be present, background sounds might be distracting or overwhelming, room temperature might impact your physical comfort, or specific scents might be either arousing or off-putting.

Temporal sensory needs recognize that your sensory preferences and tolerances change based on stress levels, energy state, hormonal cycles, and overall stimulation load from the day. You might need different types of touch or environmental conditions at different times, even within the same relationship.

Communication about sensory preferences becomes essential for satisfying physical intimacy. This includes expressing what types of touch feel good versus uncomfortable, explaining how environmental factors affect your experience, communicating when you need sensory breaks during intimate moments, or describing what helps you feel physically comfortable and present.

Jennifer's sensory accommodation process demonstrates effective strategies. She and her partner created a bedroom environment that supported her sensory needs—soft lighting options, comfortable room temperature, and minimal visual distractions. They developed simple signals for communicating comfort levels during intimate moments and established that requesting sensory adjustments was normal rather than rejecting.

Timing considerations acknowledge that your capacity for sensory-intensive experiences varies throughout days, weeks, and months. You might feel more open to touch after calming activities, need different types of physical connection after high-stimulation days, or require longer warm-up periods to feel comfortable with intimate touch.

Managing Social Energy in Couple Relationships

Romantic relationships require significant social energy even when you're with someone you love deeply. Understanding and managing this energy expenditure prevents relationship burnout while maintaining the connection and intimacy that partnerships require for long-term success.

Social energy assessment helps you understand how different relationship activities affect your energy levels. Casual conversations might feel restorative, while relationship processing discussions might be draining. Date nights might be energizing or exhausting depending on the activity and environment.

Energy budgeting for relationship activities ensures you have sufficient resources for maintaining connection while meeting other life demands. This might involve scheduling relationship conversations during high-energy times, planning simpler activities during low-energy periods, or building recovery time after socially demanding relationship events.

Parallel presence offers opportunities for connection that don't require active social engagement. You might enjoy reading in the same room, working on separate projects while physically near each other, or engaging in activities that involve shared focus rather than conversation.

Recovery time needs after social activities affect your availability for relationship interaction. You might need solitude after work before engaging in couple conversations, require quiet time after social events before processing the experience together, or benefit from low-stimulation activities when your social energy feels depleted.

Maria's energy management system illustrates effective strategies. She and her partner established "parallel time" each evening—sitting together while engaging in separate activities—before having conversation-focused connection. They scheduled relationship discussions for weekend mornings when her social energy felt highest and created signals for communicating when she needed social space without it reflecting relationship problems.

Navigating Mixed Neurotype Relationship Dynamics

Autistic-neurotypical relationships have unique strengths and challenges that differ from either same-neurotype partnerships. Understanding these dynamics helps you leverage the benefits while addressing potential areas of misunderstanding or conflict.

Complementary strengths often emerge in mixed neurotype relationships. Your detail-oriented thinking might balance your partner's big-picture perspective, your direct communication might help them express needs more clearly, your routine preferences might provide stability they appreciate, or your deep interests might introduce them to new areas of knowledge.

Different social needs require negotiation and accommodation from both partners. You might prefer smaller gatherings while they enjoy large parties, need advance notice for social plans while they prefer spontaneous invitations, or require recovery time after social events while they feel energized by them.

Processing style differences affect how you approach decisions, conflicts, and daily planning as a couple. You might need time to think through options while they process verbally, prefer structured problem-solving approaches while they work through issues emotionally, or want detailed information while they're comfortable with general plans.

Emotional expression variations can create misunderstanding when partners interpret differences as relationship problems rather than neurological variations. Your way of showing affection might differ from neurotypical expectations, your response to stress might look different from theirs, or your excitement about topics might be more intense than they're accustomed to experiencing.

Rachel's dynamic navigation shows successful approaches. She and her neurotypical partner identified their different strengths—her planning abilities and his flexibility—and divided household responsibilities accordingly. They developed systems for accommodating both their social needs and created appreciation practices for their different perspectives rather than trying to change each other.

Couples Therapy Considerations

Professional support can be beneficial for mixed neurotype couples, but finding therapists who understand autism in women and neurodiversity-affirming approaches requires careful selection and clear communication about your needs.

Therapist selection criteria should include experience with autism in adults, understanding of neurodiversity and mixed neurotype relationships, willingness to learn about your specific presentation if they lack extensive autism experience, and commitment to strength-based rather than deficit-focused approaches.

Therapy goals might include improving communication between different neurotypes, developing accommodation strategies that work for both partners, processing relationship conflicts through neurodiversity-informed perspectives, or building appreciation for different cognitive and emotional styles.

Avoid conversion-focused approaches that attempt to make you more neurotypical or treat your autistic traits as relationship problems to eliminate. Effective couples therapy for mixed neurotype relationships focuses on mutual understanding and accommodation rather than changing fundamental neurological differences.

Preparation strategies help you get maximum benefit from couples therapy sessions. Prepare specific examples of communication challenges or accommodation needs, identify relationship strengths to build upon, clarify your goals for therapy, or gather information about autism in women to share with therapists who need education.

Amanda's therapy experience demonstrates effective approaches. She and her partner found a therapist who specialized in neurodiversity and spent initial sessions educating the therapist about her specific autism presentation. They focused on developing communication strategies that honored both their styles and created accommodation plans for common relationship challenges.

Building Understanding and Accommodation

Successful mixed neurotype relationships require ongoing commitment to mutual understanding and accommodation from both partners. This process involves continuous learning, adjustment, and appreciation for different ways of experiencing and interacting with the world.

Mutual education helps both partners understand how autism affects daily life and relationship dynamics. This might involve your partner learning about sensory processing differences, executive function challenges, or communication preferences while you learn about neurotypical social expectations, emotional expression patterns, or decision-making processes.

Accommodation planning develops specific strategies for supporting both partners' needs in practical daily situations. This might include environmental modifications that support your sensory needs, communication agreements that honor different processing styles, social planning that considers both your energy patterns, or conflict resolution approaches that work for different cognitive styles.

Appreciation practices build positive relationship dynamics by recognizing and celebrating neurological differences as sources of strength rather than challenges to overcome. This might involve acknowledging how your attention to detail improves household organization, appreciating your partner's social skills in challenging situations, or celebrating how your different perspectives create more complete solutions to problems.

Regular check-ins maintain accommodation strategies and address new challenges as they arise. Relationships change over time, and accommodation needs might shift with life circumstances, stress levels, or increased self-understanding. Schedule regular conversations about what's working well and what might need adjustment.

Conflict resolution frameworks that account for different communication and processing styles prevent minor misunderstandings from becoming major relationship problems. This might include using written communication for complex issues, taking breaks during heated discussions to allow processing time, or developing structured approaches for working through disagreements.

The Path Forward Together

Mixed neurotype relationships offer unique opportunities for growth, understanding, and connection when both partners approach autism as a difference to accommodate rather than a problem to solve. Your autism brings specific strengths to your relationship—honesty, loyalty, attention to detail, and deep capacity for interest and care—that can create profound intimacy and partnership.

The accommodation process works both ways in healthy relationships. While your partner learns to support your sensory needs and communication preferences, you also learn to understand their social and emotional patterns. This mutual adjustment creates relationships based on genuine understanding rather than assumptions about how people should think or feel.

Long-term success in mixed neurotype relationships depends on maintaining curiosity about each other's experiences, continuing to develop accommodation strategies as life changes, and building appreciation for the unique perspectives that different neurotypes bring to partnership. Your autism doesn't make relationships harder—it makes them different, and different can be extraordinary when embraced fully.

Chapter 8: Parenting While Autistic

- Motherhood Through an Autistic Lens

Autistic mothers bring unique strengths and face specific challenges that differ significantly from neurotypical parenting experiences. Your intense attention to detail, pattern recognition abilities, and deep capacity for special interests can become powerful parenting tools, while sensory overwhelm and executive function differences require accommodation strategies that support both you and your children.

The mythology of perfect motherhood doesn't account for neurological differences, often leaving autistic mothers feeling inadequate when standard parenting advice doesn't work for their families. Dr. Michelle Sutton's research reveals that autistic mothers often excel at creating structured, predictable environments that benefit all children while struggling with chaotic social situations that other parents handle easily (34). Understanding these patterns helps you parent from your strengths rather than fighting against your neurology.

Recognizing Autism in Your Children

Autism has strong genetic components, meaning your children may also be autistic. Your personal experience with autism provides unique advantages for recognizing and supporting neurodivergent traits in your children, though it can also create emotional complexity as you process your own childhood experiences simultaneously.

Early recognition signs in children often differ from textbook descriptions, particularly in girls. You might notice intense interests that seem advanced for their age, unusual sensory reactions or preferences, social interaction patterns that remind you of your own childhood, or communication styles that feel familiar from your autistic experience.

Trust your observations even when professionals dismiss your concerns. Your lived experience with autism provides insights that many healthcare providers lack. You understand what masking looks like in children, recognize subtle sensory sensitivities, and identify social challenges that might not be obvious to neurotypical observers.

Gender differences in autism presentation mean that daughters might be particularly difficult for others to identify as autistic. You might recognize female autism patterns— like your daughter's elaborate fantasy play, her intense friendship dynamics, or her tendency to mimic others—that get dismissed as typical girl behavior by teachers or physicians.

Multiple children considerations become complex when you have both autistic and neurotypical children. You might notice marked differences in their development, communication styles, or sensory responses. Managing different neurotypes within one family requires flexible approaches that support each child's unique needs.

Karen's recognition journey illustrates these dynamics. She noticed that her 4-year-old daughter arranged toys in complex patterns, became distressed when routines changed unexpectedly, and preferred parallel play to interactive games. While teachers dismissed these behaviors as normal preschooler development, Karen recognized familiar autism patterns and pursued evaluation despite professional resistance.

Documentation strategies help you track patterns and communicate concerns to professionals. Keep notes about your child's sensory reactions, social interactions, communication development, and behavioral patterns. Video recordings can capture subtle behaviors that might not occur during brief professional observations.

Using Your Autistic Traits as Parenting Strengths

Your autism brings specific advantages to parenting that often go unrecognized in parenting literature focused on neurotypical experiences. These strengths can be developed and leveraged to create exceptional parenting approaches that benefit your entire family.

Pattern recognition abilities help you identify your children's individual needs, preferences, and developmental patterns more quickly than many parents. You might notice that your child focuses better after physical activity, becomes overwhelmed in specific environments, or learns more effectively through particular teaching methods.

Attention to detail allows you to track important information about your children's health, development, and educational needs. You might notice subtle changes in behavior that indicate illness, recognize learning patterns that teachers miss, or identify environmental factors that affect your child's functioning.

Research skills developed through pursuing special interests can be applied to understanding child development, educational options, medical needs, or behavioral strategies. Your ability to become an expert in areas that interest you serves your children well when applied to parenting topics.

Structured thinking helps you create consistent routines, organized environments, and predictable family systems that benefit all children, particularly those who are also neurodivergent. Your natural tendency toward organization and planning can create stability that supports healthy child development.

Direct communication with your children builds authentic relationships based on honesty and clear expectations. Your straightforward style can be refreshing for children who appreciate knowing exactly what's expected of them and why certain rules exist.

Lisa's strength utilization demonstrates these advantages. Her pattern recognition helped her identify that her son learned better through visual methods before teachers recognized this need. Her research abilities led her to find educational resources that dramatically improved his academic performance. Her structured approach created household routines that reduced chaos and increased everyone's sense of security.

Managing Sensory Overwhelm in Family Environments

Families create complex sensory environments that can be overwhelming for autistic mothers. Children's needs, household activities, and family life generate constant sensory input that requires management strategies to prevent overload while maintaining family functioning.

Household sensory planning involves creating environments that support your sensory needs while accommodating family activities. This might include designated quiet spaces where you can retreat when overwhelmed, lighting modifications that reduce sensory stress, sound management strategies for noisy family activities, or organization systems that reduce visual chaos.

Activity modification adapts family routines to support your sensory processing needs. This might involve choosing restaurants based on acoustic levels and lighting, planning outdoor activities during times that work for your sensory system, modifying holiday celebrations to reduce overwhelming elements, or creating alternative traditions that work better for your family's needs.

Recovery strategies help you manage sensory overload when it occurs during family time. This might include brief retreats to quiet spaces during busy family activities, using sensory tools like noise-canceling headphones during children's playtime, or scheduling regular breaks during demanding family events.

Family communication about sensory needs helps children understand and support your requirements while learning about their own sensory preferences. Explain why certain environments are challenging for you, teach children to recognize signs that you need sensory breaks, and create family signals for communicating sensory overwhelm.

Environmental modifications might include sound-absorbing materials in play areas, dimmable lighting throughout the house, organized storage systems that reduce visual clutter, or designated spaces for different types of family activities. These changes often benefit the entire family while specifically supporting your sensory needs.

Jennifer's management system illustrates effective strategies. She created a quiet reading corner where she could retreat during overwhelming moments, established "quiet time" each afternoon when the whole family engaged in calm activities, used noise-canceling headphones during children's loud play, and modified family outings to include sensory-friendly options.

Creating Structure and Routine That Works

Autistic mothers often excel at creating structured family environments, but the key lies in developing flexible systems that support everyone's needs rather than rigid schedules that create stress when disrupted.

Routine development should account for both your need for predictability and your children's developmental requirements. This might involve consistent morning and evening routines that provide structure, weekly schedules that balance planned activities with flexible time, or seasonal routines that adapt to changing family needs throughout the year.

Visual scheduling helps the entire family understand expectations and reduces the executive function demands on you for constant family coordination. Use visual calendars that show family activities, create daily routine charts that children can follow independently, or establish visual systems for tracking family responsibilities and expectations.

Flexibility within structure prevents routine rigidity while maintaining beneficial predictability. Build buffer time into schedules for unexpected delays, create backup plans for common disruptions, or establish "plan B" activities that can replace original plans when necessary.

Family systems that distribute responsibilities reduce the cognitive load on you while teaching children important life skills. This might involve age-appropriate chores that children can manage independently, family meeting systems for discussing household needs, or rotation systems for family responsibilities.

Special interest integration involves incorporating your areas of expertise and passion into family activities. This might mean using your knowledge of specific topics for educational family projects, sharing your interests with children who express curiosity, or finding ways to connect family activities to subjects that energize you.

Rachel's system development shows these principles in action. She created visual schedules for morning and evening routines, established weekly family meetings for planning activities, built flexibility into schedules by using time blocks rather than exact times, and integrated her special interest in gardening into family activities that taught children about nature and responsibility.

Advocating for Neurodivergent Children

Your experience as an autistic woman provides unique advantages for advocating effectively for neurodivergent children in educational and social settings. Your understanding of autism, combined with your parental authority, creates powerful advocacy positions.

Educational advocacy involves working with schools to ensure appropriate support for your neurodivergent children. This might include requesting evaluations for special education services, advocating for classroom accommodations that support learning, communicating with teachers about effective strategies, or ensuring that school plans address your child's specific needs.

Medical advocacy helps ensure your children receive appropriate healthcare that accounts for their neurodivergent needs. This might involve finding healthcare providers who understand autism, preparing children for medical appointments to reduce anxiety, advocating for accommodations during medical procedures, or ensuring that medical recommendations account for sensory and communication differences.

Social advocacy involves helping your children navigate social situations while building self-advocacy skills. This might include teaching them about their neurodivergent traits, helping them identify and communicate their needs, advocating with other parents for inclusive social activities, or creating social opportunities that work well for neurodivergent children.

Self-advocacy skill development prepares your children to advocate for themselves as they grow older. This involves teaching them about their strengths and challenges, helping them develop language for explaining their needs, practicing advocacy skills in low-stakes situations, or modeling effective advocacy through your own behavior.

Documentation and organization supports effective advocacy by maintaining records of your children's needs, interventions, and progress. Keep organized files of evaluation reports, maintain communication logs with schools and providers, document successful strategies and accommodations, or create portfolios that demonstrate your children's abilities and growth.

Maria's advocacy approach demonstrates effective strategies. She maintained detailed documentation of her daughter's educational needs, developed collaborative relationships with teachers by sharing successful strategies, organized with other parents to advocate for sensory-friendly classroom environments, and taught her daughter to communicate her own accommodation needs as she got older.

Self-Care Strategies for Autistic Mothers

Parenting as an autistic woman requires intentional self-care strategies that account for your specific neurological needs while managing the demands of family life. These aren't luxuries—they're necessary supports that enable sustainable parenting.

Energy management involves recognizing and planning for the high cognitive and sensory demands of parenting. This might include scheduling demanding parenting tasks during your peak energy times, building recovery periods into daily schedules, or identifying which parenting activities are most draining for you personally.

Sensory self-care addresses the reality that family life creates constant sensory input that can become overwhelming. This might involve using noise-canceling headphones during children's loud activities, creating sensory retreats within your home, or scheduling regular breaks in low-stimulation environments.

Social energy conservation recognizes that parenting involves significant social interaction that can be exhausting. This might include limiting additional social commitments during busy family periods, scheduling recovery time after social parenting events, or finding ways to connect with other parents that feel less draining.

Special interest maintenance ensures that you continue engaging with topics and activities that bring you joy and regulation. This might involve scheduling regular time for your interests, finding ways to share interests with family members, or using special interests as stress relief during challenging parenting periods.

Support system development creates networks that understand and accommodate your autistic parenting needs. This might include connecting with other neurodivergent parents, finding babysitters who understand your family's needs, or building relationships with professionals who support your parenting approach.

Professional self-care might include therapy with providers who understand autism in women, medical care that accounts for your sensory and communication needs, or consultation with autism specialists about family challenges.

Susan's self-care system illustrates comprehensive approaches. She scheduled daily quiet time during her children's rest periods, maintained weekly time for her special interests, connected with other autistic mothers through online support groups, used noise-canceling headphones during overwhelming family activities, and worked with a therapist who understood autism in women and parenting challenges.

Building Support Networks

Isolation is common among autistic mothers, but building support networks specifically designed to understand and accommodate your needs creates essential resources for both daily support and crisis management.

Neurodivergent parent communities provide understanding and practical advice from parents who share similar experiences. These might include online support groups for autistic mothers, local meetups for neurodivergent families, or social media communities focused on autism and parenting.

Professional support networks include service providers who understand autism in women and support your parenting approach. This might involve autism-informed therapists, pediatric providers who understand neurodivergent children, or educational advocates who support inclusive approaches.

Family support systems help extended family members understand and support your autistic parenting needs. This might involve educating grandparents about autism in women, explaining your children's neurodivergent traits to family members, or setting boundaries around family gatherings that don't accommodate your needs.

Practical support networks provide concrete assistance with parenting tasks and family management. This might include childcare providers who understand neurodivergent children, carpools with families who accommodate different needs, or household help that reduces sensory and executive function demands.

Emergency support planning creates systems for managing crises when your usual supports aren't available. This might involve backup childcare for autism burnout periods, emergency contact lists for family crises, or support protocols for managing overwhelming family situations.

Amy's network development shows effective strategies. She connected with other autistic mothers through social media groups, found a pediatrician who understood sensory processing differences, educated her mother about autism in women to improve family support, established regular childcare with a provider who understood her children's needs, and created emergency plans for managing overwhelming periods.

Growth Through Authentic Parenting

Parenting as an autistic woman requires courage to parent authentically rather than attempting to conform to neurotypical parenting expectations. This authenticity often creates stronger family relationships and teaches children valuable lessons about acceptance and accommodation.

Your autism brings specific strengths to parenting that can create exceptional family experiences when embraced fully. Your attention to detail, deep capacity for interest and care, and structured thinking often translate into parenting approaches that support healthy child development while honoring everyone's neurological differences.

The challenges you face as an autistic mother are real and require accommodation, but they don't diminish your capacity for effective, loving parenting. Creating support systems, developing self-care strategies, and building on your autistic strengths allows you to parent sustainably while maintaining your own wellbeing.

Your children benefit from seeing authentic self-advocacy, accommodation strategies, and appreciation for neurological differences modeled in their daily family life. This exposure often creates more accepting, flexible individuals who understand and celebrate human diversity.

Chapter 9: Building Authentic Friendships

- Social Connection Strategies

Friendship for autistic women often feels like trying to solve a puzzle with missing pieces—you understand the general concept but struggle with the unspoken rules, energy demands, and social expectations that seem to come naturally to others. Building authentic friendships requires abandoning neurotypical friendship models and creating connections based on genuine compatibility, shared interests, and mutual accommodation.

Traditional friendship advice assumes neurotypical social processing and energy patterns, often leaving autistic women feeling inadequate when these strategies fail spectacularly. Dr. Chloe Rothschild's research shows that autistic women who build friendships around shared interests and direct communication often report higher satisfaction and longer-lasting relationships than those attempting to follow conventional social scripts (35).

Why Traditional Friendship Advice Falls Short

Mainstream friendship guidance assumes social skills and energy patterns that don't match autistic experiences. These approaches often backfire for autistic women, creating exhaustion and inauthenticity rather than meaningful connection.

Small talk expectations dominate conventional friendship advice, suggesting that casual conversation builds relationships gradually. For autistic women, small talk often feels meaningless, draining, and difficult to sustain. You might prefer jumping directly into substantive conversations about topics that genuinely interest both people.

Spontaneous social activities get promoted as essential for friendship development, but unexpected plans can trigger anxiety and overwhelm for autistic individuals. You might need advance notice to prepare mentally, time to arrange your environment and energy for social interaction, or structured activities that provide conversation frameworks.

Reciprocal social energy assumptions underlying traditional advice don't account for autistic social processing differences. While neurotypical friends might energize each other through social interaction, you might find that even enjoyable socializing requires recovery time afterward.

Nonverbal communication emphasis in friendship building ignores the reality that many autistic women struggle to read or produce expected nonverbal cues. Advice about "reading body language" or "picking up social hints" can feel impossible when your brain doesn't process these signals naturally.

Frequency expectations about friendship contact often don't match autistic patterns. You might prefer deeper, less frequent interactions rather than daily casual contact, or you might need friendship patterns that account for sensory overload and social energy cycles.

Sarah's traditional approach failure illustrates these mismatches. She followed advice about joining social groups and making small talk, which left her exhausted and feeling more isolated than before. She forced herself to attend frequent social gatherings, which led to autistic burnout. Only when she began seeking connections through shared interests did she find genuine friendships that energized rather than drained her.

Finding Your Tribe Among Neurodivergent Women

Connecting with other neurodivergent women often provides the foundation for friendships that truly understand and accommodate your needs while offering mutual support and genuine compatibility.

Shared neurological experiences create immediate understanding that doesn't require extensive explanation or justification. You might find that conversations about sensory experiences, executive function challenges, or masking fatigue feel validating and normal rather than requiring constant translation for neurotypical understanding.

Communication style compatibility emerges naturally with other autistic women who often prefer direct communication, deeper conversations, and honest emotional expression. You might discover that conversations flow more naturally when both people share similar communication preferences and processing styles.

Accommodation understanding develops more easily with friends who have their own neurological differences and understand the need for environmental modifications, energy management, and flexible social expectations. These friendships often involve mutual accommodation that benefits everyone.

Reduced masking demands allow you to express your authentic self more freely with friends who understand and appreciate autistic traits. You might find that stimming, discussing special interests enthusiastically, or requesting sensory accommodations feels natural rather than embarrassing.

Online communities provide accessible ways to connect with other neurodivergent women without the sensory and social demands of in-person interaction. You might build friendships through autism-focused social media groups, forums, or virtual meetups that allow connection from your own sensory-comfortable environment.

Local neurodivergent groups offer opportunities for in-person connection with people who understand your experiences. These might include autism support groups, neurodivergent professional networks, or special interest groups that attract neurodivergent individuals.

Jennifer's tribe discovery demonstrates this process. After years of struggling to maintain neurotypical friendships, she joined an online autism support group where she connected with women who shared similar experiences. These connections led to local meetups, regular video calls, and friendships that required no explanation or accommodation requests—the understanding was built into the foundation.

Managing Social Energy and Preventing Burnout

Friendship requires social energy investment, but autistic women need strategies for managing these demands without reaching burnout. Understanding your social energy patterns allows you to maintain friendships sustainably over time.

Social energy assessment helps you understand which friendship activities energize versus drain you. You might find that structured activities with clear purposes feel less demanding than unstructured social time, or that certain friends require less energy to interact with than others.

Energy budgeting for social activities ensures you maintain sufficient resources for work, family, and personal needs while investing in friendships. This might involve limiting social commitments during high-stress periods, scheduling recovery time after demanding social events, or choosing friendship activities based on your available energy.

Batching social activities can be more efficient than spreading interactions throughout the week. You might prefer scheduling multiple social interactions in one day followed by recovery time, or grouping similar types of social activities together to minimize cognitive switching demands.

Virtual connection options provide ways to maintain friendships that require less sensory and social energy. You might use video calls, messaging apps, or online games to stay connected with friends when in-person interaction feels overwhelming.

Boundary communication with friends about your social energy needs prevents misunderstandings and supports long-term friendship sustainability. This might involve explaining why you need advance notice for plans, requesting modifications to social activities, or communicating when you need social space without it reflecting friendship problems.

Recovery protocols help you return to baseline functioning after social activities. This might include scheduling quiet time after social events, engaging in self-soothing activities, or allowing extra time for processing social interactions.

Lisa's energy management illustrates effective strategies. She discovered that she could handle more social interaction when she scheduled activities during her peak energy times, limited herself to one major social event per week, and communicated her energy patterns to close friends who began offering lower-energy connection options during busy periods.

Navigating Small Talk and Social Expectations

While you can't eliminate small talk entirely from social interactions, you can develop strategies for managing these exchanges while steering conversations toward more meaningful territory.

Small talk scripts provide frameworks for managing brief social exchanges without depleting cognitive resources. Develop standard responses to common questions, practice transitioning from surface topics to deeper conversations, or prepare conversation starters that move beyond weather and pleasantries.

Transition strategies help you move from obligatory social exchanges to conversations that genuinely interest you. This might involve asking follow-up questions that reveal deeper topics, sharing something personal to encourage reciprocal sharing, or directly expressing interest in learning more about specific aspects of what someone has shared.

Time-limited approaches to small talk prevent these interactions from becoming overwhelming. You might set mental time limits for casual conversation before steering toward deeper topics, or use small talk as a brief warm-up before transitioning to more substantive discussion.

Interest-based redirects allow you to acknowledge social expectations while moving toward topics that energize you. This might involve connecting casual topics to your areas of expertise, asking questions that reveal others' interests, or sharing enthusiasm about related topics that genuinely engage you.

Energy-conserving strategies help you participate in expected social exchanges without depleting resources needed for meaningful conversation. This might involve using standard phrases that require minimal cognitive effort, preparing conversation topics in advance, or choosing social environments that support rather than challenge your social processing.

Maria's navigation approach shows practical implementation. She developed a mental toolkit of conversation transitions that helped her move from small talk to topics she enjoyed discussing, practiced asking questions that revealed others' genuine interests, and gave herself permission to be honest about preferring deeper conversations rather than apologizing for her communication style.

Creating Deeper Connections Through Shared Interests

Your special interests and areas of expertise can become powerful foundations for authentic friendships when you connect with people who share your enthusiasm or appreciate your knowledge.

Interest-based communities provide natural opportunities to meet people who share your passions and understand the depth of engagement that characterizes autistic interests. These might include hobby groups, professional organizations, online forums, or classes related to your areas of expertise.

Teaching and learning dynamics often emerge naturally in interest-based friendships, creating mutual value and connection. You might find satisfaction in sharing your expertise while learning from others' knowledge, creating relationships based on genuine curiosity and appreciation for each other's contributions.

Project-based connections provide structured frameworks for building friendships around shared goals and interests. This might involve collaborative creative projects, volunteer work for causes you care about, or participating in group activities that have clear purposes and outcomes.

Expertise appreciation creates opportunities for friendships with people who value your deep knowledge even if they don't share your specific interests. You might connect with individuals who appreciate learning from your expertise while offering their own knowledge in different areas.

Passionate conversation opportunities emerge when you find people who enjoy enthusiastic discussions about topics that genuinely matter to you. These conversations often feel energizing rather than draining because they align with your natural communication style and areas of strength.

Mentorship relationships can develop in either direction—you might mentor others in your areas of expertise or learn from people whose knowledge complements your interests. These relationships often feel more comfortable because they have clear purposes and established frameworks for interaction.

Rachel's interest-based approach demonstrates these strategies. Her passion for historical textiles led her to join a fiber arts guild where she connected with people who appreciated her extensive knowledge. These relationships developed naturally through shared projects, teaching opportunities, and collaborative learning experiences that felt energizing rather than socially demanding.

Setting Boundaries in Friendships

Healthy friendships require clear boundaries that protect your energy, honor your needs, and maintain the sustainability of your relationships over time. These boundaries often need to be more explicit than in neurotypical friendships.

Communication boundaries establish how and when you prefer to interact with friends. This might involve expressing preferences for text versus phone communication, requesting advance notice for plans, or explaining your need for processing time before responding to complex emotional situations.

Energy boundaries protect your social and emotional resources while maintaining friendship connections. This might include limiting the frequency of social interactions, requesting modifications to draining activities, or communicating when you need social space without it indicating relationship problems.

Sensory boundaries ensure that friendship activities support rather than overwhelm your sensory system. This might involve choosing restaurants based on acoustic levels, requesting specific seating arrangements during group activities, or explaining your need for environmental accommodations.

Emotional boundaries protect your capacity to process and respond to friends' emotional needs while maintaining your own stability. This might include communicating your availability for emotional support, requesting written communication for complex emotional topics, or explaining your processing style for emotional conversations.

Time boundaries help you balance friendship investments with other life demands and energy requirements. This might involve scheduling regular but limited contact, explaining your need for advance planning, or setting realistic expectations about your availability during high-stress periods.

Accommodation boundaries clarify which adjustments you need from friends while identifying what accommodations you can reasonably provide in return. This creates mutual understanding about the support each person needs for successful friendship.

Jennifer's boundary development illustrates effective approaches. She learned to communicate her need for advance notice about social plans, explained her preference for structured activities over unstructured hanging out, and established regular check-ins with close friends about what was working well and what needed adjustment in their friendship patterns.

Quality Over Quantity in Social Relationships

Autistic women often thrive with fewer but deeper friendships rather than large social networks that require extensive energy maintenance. This approach aligns with your processing style and social energy patterns.

Deep connection preferences often characterize autistic friendship patterns. You might prefer having thorough conversations with one person rather than brief interactions with many people, or find satisfaction in developing expertise about your friends' lives, interests, and experiences.

Loyalty and consistency often mark autistic friendship styles. You might form intense attachments to friends who understand and appreciate you, maintain friendships over long periods despite geographic or life changes, or invest heavily in relationships that feel authentic and mutual.

Quality indicators help you identify friendships worth investing your limited social energy in. These might include friends who appreciate your authentic self, relationships that feel energizing rather than draining, people who accommodate your needs without making you feel burdensome, or connections that allow mutual support and understanding.

Maintenance strategies for quality friendships often differ from neurotypical approaches. You might prefer less frequent but more meaningful contact, scheduled regular check-ins rather than spontaneous communication, or structured activities that provide frameworks for connection.

Energy investment decisions become crucial when you have limited social resources. You might choose to invest deeply in fewer relationships rather than maintaining many superficial connections, or prioritize friendships that provide mutual support and understanding over those that require constant accommodation.

Social network optimization involves arranging your friendships to support your overall wellbeing and life goals. This might include having different friends for different types of support, maintaining some relationships primarily online, or creating friend groups around shared interests or activities.

Amy's quality approach demonstrates these principles. Rather than trying to maintain a large social circle, she focused on developing three close friendships with women who understood her autism, shared her interests, and appreciated her direct communication style. These relationships provided more satisfaction and support than the larger but superficial social network she had previously attempted to maintain.

Maintaining Long-Distance and Virtual Friendships

Technology creates opportunities for maintaining meaningful friendships that don't require the sensory demands and energy expenditure of frequent in-person interaction. These relationships can be particularly satisfying for autistic women.

Digital communication advantages often align well with autistic communication preferences. You might find that written communication allows more thoughtful responses, video calls provide visual connection without sensory overwhelm, or online activities create structured ways to spend time together.

Asynchronous interaction benefits accommodate different processing speeds and energy patterns. You might prefer messaging apps that allow responding when you have mental resources available, email exchanges that permit thoughtful responses, or voice messages that combine personal connection with flexible timing.

Virtual activity options provide ways to share experiences with long-distance friends. This might include online games that create shared activities, virtual museum tours or learning experiences, or watching movies together through streaming platforms.

Scheduled connection patterns help maintain consistency in long-distance friendships. You might establish regular video call times, plan virtual activities in advance, or create ongoing projects that provide reasons for regular contact.

Mixed interaction approaches combine various communication methods based on energy levels and circumstances. You might use quick texts for maintaining contact, longer emails for deeper communication, and scheduled calls for more personal connection.

Technology accommodation strategies help you use digital tools effectively for friendship maintenance. This might involve using noise-canceling headphones during video calls, adjusting screen settings to reduce visual stress, or choosing communication platforms that work well with your sensory needs.

Susan's virtual friendship success illustrates these strategies. She maintained close friendships with autistic women across the country through regular video calls, shared online activities, and ongoing message exchanges that allowed deep conversation without the sensory demands of in-person interaction.

Building Community Through Authentic Connection

Creating authentic friendships often leads to building broader communities of understanding and support. Your willingness to be genuine about your autism creates space for others to be authentic about their own differences and challenges.

Autism advocacy through friendship occurs naturally when you model authentic self-expression and accommodation requests. Your friends learn about autism through your experiences, often becoming advocates and allies who support broader autism acceptance.

Community creation happens when you connect multiple neurodivergent individuals who share similar experiences and needs. You might facilitate introductions between autistic friends, organize gatherings that accommodate multiple people's sensory needs, or create social opportunities designed around shared interests.

Mentorship opportunities emerge as you gain experience building successful autistic friendships. You might support newly diagnosed women in developing social connections, share strategies that have worked for you, or provide guidance about navigating neurotypical social expectations.

Family education occurs when your authentic friendships demonstrate positive autism representation to family members who may have misconceptions about autistic capabilities. Your successful relationships provide evidence that autism doesn't prevent meaningful connection.

Professional influence can develop when your friendship experiences inform your work or volunteer activities. You might use your understanding of autistic social needs in professional settings, advocate for inclusive social practices, or contribute to autism research and understanding.

The Rewards of Authentic Connection

Building genuine friendships as an autistic woman requires courage to abandon neurotypical social expectations and create relationships based on mutual understanding, shared interests, and accommodation. These authentic connections often provide deeper satisfaction than relationships built on social performance.

Your direct communication style, loyalty, and deep capacity for interest create unique friendship strengths when matched with compatible individuals. The energy you invest in building authentic relationships returns in the form of support, understanding, and genuine connection that sustains you through life's challenges.

The friendships you build by being authentically autistic contribute to broader social understanding and acceptance. Each genuine relationship you form demonstrates that autism doesn't prevent meaningful connection—it simply requires different approaches and mutual accommodation.

Your willingness to seek authentic rather than convenient relationships models self-advocacy and authentic living for others, both autistic and neurotypical. These relationships become foundations for community, support, and personal growth that honor your neurodivergent identity while meeting your genuine social needs.

Wrapping Up Your Social Journey

Friendship as an autistic woman looks different from neurotypical social experiences, but different doesn't mean less valuable or meaningful. Your approach to building connections through shared interests, direct communication, and mutual understanding often creates relationships with exceptional depth and loyalty.

The energy you conserve by abandoning ineffective neurotypical social strategies becomes available for nurturing relationships that truly support and appreciate you. This shift from quantity to quality often results in more satisfying social lives that align with your energy patterns and communication preferences.

Your success in building authentic friendships provides a model for other autistic women who may struggle with conventional social advice. The community you create through genuine connection contributes to broader autism acceptance and understanding while providing personal support and belonging.

Essential Insights From This Section:

- Traditional friendship advice often fails autistic women because it assumes neurotypical social processing and energy patterns

- Connecting with other neurodivergent women provides natural understanding and reduces masking demands in friendships

- Managing social energy through strategic planning and boundary setting prevents friendship-related burnout

- Building friendships around shared interests creates natural foundations for authentic connection and mutual appreciation

- Quality relationships often provide more satisfaction than large social networks for autistic women

- Virtual and long-distance friendships can be particularly sustainable and meaningful when managed thoughtfully

- Authentic relationships contribute to broader autism acceptance while providing personal support and community

Chapter 10: Workplace Success Strategies

- Professional Life Navigation

The modern workplace wasn't designed with autistic women in mind, yet you bring exceptional strengths that can drive professional success when properly supported and understood. Your attention to detail, pattern recognition abilities, and deep focus can be career assets, but navigating office politics, sensory challenges, and disclosure decisions requires strategic planning and self-advocacy skills that most career guides never address.

Dr. Sarah Cassidy's workplace research reveals that autistic women often excel in their core job functions while struggling with ancillary social demands like networking events, team lunches, and informal communication expectations (36). Understanding this pattern helps you focus on building career strategies that leverage your strengths while managing the aspects of work that feel most challenging.

Disclosure Decisions That Protect and Advance Your Career

Deciding when, how, and to whom to disclose your autism at work represents one of the most complex professional decisions you'll face. This choice affects your access to accommodations, colleagues' perceptions, and your long-term career trajectory in ways that require careful consideration.

Timing considerations significantly impact how your disclosure is received and what support you can access. Disclosing during the interview process protects you legally but might affect hiring decisions despite legal protections. Waiting until after you're established in a role provides job security but might make requesting accommodations more challenging.

Strategic disclosure approaches allow you to share information gradually based on your comfort level and workplace culture. You might start by discussing specific accommodation needs without mentioning autism, then provide more context if additional support becomes necessary. This approach lets you test workplace responsiveness before full disclosure.

Audience selection matters significantly when you decide to disclose. Human resources departments are legally required to maintain confidentiality and process accommodation requests, while direct supervisors might need to understand your needs to provide effective management. Colleagues require different information than administrators.

Documentation preparation supports your disclosure by providing official evidence of your diagnosis and specific accommodation needs. This might include letters from healthcare providers, documentation of successful accommodations from previous positions, or detailed explanations of how specific supports improve your job performance.

Legal protection understanding helps you make informed disclosure decisions. The Americans with Disabilities Act provides employment protections, but understanding exactly what this means for your situation requires research or consultation with disability rights organizations or employment attorneys.

Jennifer's disclosure strategy illustrates thoughtful approaches. She worked successfully in her marketing role for six months before disclosing her autism to her supervisor. She prepared a letter explaining her diagnosis, documented specific accommodations that would improve her productivity, and emphasized how these supports would benefit the team's overall performance. Her supervisor implemented the requested accommodations without involving HR or other team members.

Requesting Accommodations Without Full Disclosure

You can access many workplace accommodations without disclosing your autism diagnosis by focusing on specific needs and their business benefits rather than underlying neurological differences.

Accommodation framing emphasizes how modifications improve your productivity and job performance rather than addressing disability-related challenges. Request noise-canceling headphones to improve focus rather than explaining auditory sensitivities. Ask for written meeting agendas to enhance preparation rather than discussing executive function differences.

Business case development connects your accommodation requests to organizational benefits. Explain how specific environmental modifications will improve your accuracy, how alternative communication methods will increase your efficiency, or how schedule modifications will optimize your contributions to team goals.

Gradual implementation allows you to test accommodations and demonstrate their effectiveness before requesting more significant modifications. Start with simple requests like preferred seating or lighting adjustments, then expand to additional accommodations as you establish credibility and workplace relationships.

Performance emphasis connects accommodation requests to demonstrated work quality and productivity improvements. Document how specific modifications enhance your output, reduce errors, or increase your capacity to take on additional responsibilities.

Specific request strategies focus on concrete modifications rather than general accommodation categories. Request permission to wear noise-canceling headphones during focused work rather than asking for "sensory accommodations." Ask for consistent meeting times rather than requesting "schedule predictability."

Universal design benefits highlight how many autism-friendly accommodations improve the workplace for multiple employees. Reduced background noise benefits many people's concentration, clear written communication improves understanding for most team members, and organized meeting structures help everyone participate more effectively.

Lisa's accommodation approach demonstrates effective strategies. She requested permission to work from a quieter area of the office to improve concentration, asked for meeting agendas 24 hours in advance to prepare effectively, and negotiated a modified schedule that avoided peak commuting times. She framed these requests around productivity improvements and demonstrated their effectiveness through measurably better work output.

Managing Workplace Social Dynamics

Office politics and workplace social expectations can be particularly challenging for autistic women, but understanding these dynamics and developing strategic responses allows you to maintain professional relationships while protecting your energy and authenticity.

Informal communication networks carry significant workplace information and influence that formal channels often miss. You might need to identify key people who share important updates, find alternative ways to access information typically shared through casual conversation, or develop relationships with colleagues who can provide social context for workplace dynamics.

Meeting participation strategies help you contribute effectively while managing social and sensory demands. This might involve preparing talking points in advance, positioning yourself in seats that minimize sensory distraction, or developing techniques for participating in discussions without dominating or withdrawing completely.

Social event navigation requires balancing relationship building with energy management. You might attend events briefly to maintain visibility, find quieter areas within social gatherings for meaningful conversations, or develop alternative ways to build colleague relationships that don't rely on large group socializing.

Email and written communication optimization can become significant professional strengths when you develop systems that work with your thinking style. Your direct communication style often translates well to written formats where clarity and precision are valued over social pleasantries.

Conflict resolution approaches might differ from neurotypical workplace expectations but can be equally effective when you understand your patterns and develop appropriate strategies. You might prefer written communication for complex disagreements, need time to process feedback before responding, or benefit from structured approaches to workplace conflicts.

Professional boundary management helps you maintain workplace relationships while protecting your energy and authenticity. This might involve limiting personal disclosure in professional relationships, developing strategies for declining social invitations diplomatically, or creating clear separations between work and personal time.

Maria's navigation system shows practical implementation. She identified two colleagues who regularly shared important informal information and built relationships with them through work-related conversations. She prepared standard talking points for common workplace discussions, attended team events for exactly 30 minutes to maintain visibility, and developed written communication templates that conveyed professionalism while matching her direct style.

Leveraging Your Autistic Strengths at Work

Your autism brings specific professional advantages that can drive career success when you understand and develop them strategically. These strengths often differentiate you from colleagues in ways that create unique value for employers.

Pattern recognition abilities allow you to identify trends, inconsistencies, and connections that others might miss.

This skill applies to data analysis, quality control, process improvement, strategic planning, or problem-solving roles where attention to patterns creates significant value.

Deep focus capabilities enable you to work on complex projects with sustained attention that produces high-quality results. This strength becomes particularly valuable in roles requiring detailed analysis, creative development, research, or any work that benefits from extended concentration periods.

Systematic thinking approaches help you develop organized, logical solutions to workplace challenges. Your tendency to create systems and processes can improve team efficiency, reduce errors, and create sustainable workflows that benefit entire organizations.

Quality attention often exceeds neurotypical standards, making you particularly valuable in roles where accuracy, precision, and thoroughness matter significantly. This might include editing, compliance work, technical documentation, or any field where errors have serious consequences.

Research and learning abilities developed through pursuing special interests often translate into exceptional professional development and expertise building. Your capacity to become deeply knowledgeable about topics relevant to your work can establish you as a subject matter expert.

Direct communication styles can be professional assets in contexts where clarity and honesty are valued over social politeness. This strength might be particularly valuable in technical fields, consulting, training, or any role where straightforward communication improves outcomes.

Rachel's strength development illustrates this process. Her pattern recognition abilities helped her identify inefficiencies in her company's client onboarding process, leading to her promotion to process improvement specialist. She leveraged her deep focus capacity to develop detailed solutions that reduced onboarding time by 40%, establishing her reputation as someone who could solve complex operational challenges.

Addressing Workplace Sensory Challenges

Professional environments often create sensory demands that can overwhelm autistic women, but strategic environmental modifications and personal management techniques can transform challenging workplaces into supportive career settings.

Environmental assessment helps you identify specific workplace sensory challenges and potential modification strategies. Note lighting levels and types throughout your workspace, assess acoustic conditions during different times and activities, evaluate air quality and temperature control, and identify visual distractions or organizational challenges.

Lighting modifications can dramatically improve workplace comfort and productivity. Request desk lamps to replace harsh overhead lighting, position your workspace to minimize computer screen glare, use blue light filtering glasses if permitted, or advocate for lighting improvements that benefit multiple employees.

Sound management strategies help you function effectively in acoustically challenging environments. Use noise-canceling headphones when permissible, request seating away from high-traffic areas or noisy equipment, advocate for quiet zones in open office environments, or develop signals with colleagues for managing noise levels during focused work.

Workspace organization creates visual calm and functional efficiency that supports your productivity. Organize your desk and computer files using systems that make sense to your brain, minimize visual clutter in your immediate workspace, create consistent storage and workflow patterns, or use tools that help maintain organization with minimal ongoing effort.

Break and recovery strategies help you manage sensory accumulation throughout the workday. Schedule brief breaks in quiet or low-stimulation areas, use lunch periods for sensory reset rather than socializing, create transition routines between different types of work activities, or develop quick regulation techniques you can use at your desk.

Clothing and personal modifications support sensory comfort throughout long workdays. Choose professional clothing based on fabric texture and fit comfort, modify or remove tags and seams that cause distraction, select footwear that provides comfort during long periods, or carry sensory tools that help with regulation when needed.

Sarah's sensory management demonstrates comprehensive approaches. She negotiated a workspace near a window with natural light, used noise-canceling headphones during focused work periods, organized her desk using color-coded systems that reduced visual chaos, scheduled 10-minute walks every two hours for sensory reset, and chose professional clothing based on comfort rather than fashion trends.

Remote Work Advocacy and Optimization

Remote work often provides ideal conditions for autistic women to excel professionally while managing sensory and social demands more effectively. Advocating for remote work opportunities and optimizing home office environments can significantly improve your career satisfaction and performance.

Remote work proposals should emphasize productivity benefits and business advantages rather than personal preferences or disability accommodations. Document how remote work might improve your output quality, reduce overhead costs for your employer, or allow you to work during optimal energy periods.

Productivity demonstration provides evidence that remote work enhances your job performance. Track metrics that show improved accuracy, increased output, better project completion rates, or enhanced availability during different work hours when you work from home.

Home office optimization creates professional environments that support your sensory and executive function needs. Design lighting systems that support your vision and comfort, control acoustic environments to match your focus requirements, organize workspace using systems that match your cognitive patterns, or establish routines that separate work and personal time effectively.

Communication strategy development addresses potential employer concerns about remote work collaboration and availability. Establish regular check-in schedules that demonstrate engagement, use technology tools that facilitate team communication, create systems for tracking and reporting work progress, or develop protocols for participating in virtual meetings effectively.

Hybrid arrangement negotiation might provide optimal balance between remote work benefits and workplace collaboration requirements. Propose schedules that allow remote work during high-focus periods while maintaining in-person presence for essential meetings, collaborative projects, or client interactions.

Professional development maintenance ensures that remote work doesn't limit your career advancement opportunities. Participate actively in virtual team meetings and training sessions, maintain visibility through regular communication with supervisors and colleagues, or seek professional development opportunities that don't require extensive travel or in-person attendance.

Amanda's remote advocacy shows successful strategies. She proposed a six-month remote work trial, documented 30% improvement in project completion rates during her first month working from home, established daily check-ins with her supervisor, and participated actively in virtual team meetings. Her success led to a permanent remote work arrangement that significantly improved her career satisfaction and performance.

Career Planning for Neurodivergent Success

Long-term career planning requires strategies that account for your autistic traits, energy patterns, and professional goals while building on your strengths and managing potential challenges proactively.

Strength-based career assessment identifies professional paths that align with your natural abilities and interests. Consider careers that utilize your pattern recognition skills, benefit from deep focus abilities, value systematic thinking approaches, or allow you to develop expertise in areas that genuinely interest you.

Energy sustainability planning ensures your career choices support long-term wellbeing while allowing professional growth. Evaluate workload patterns that match your energy cycles, consider work environments that don't require constant masking, or choose career paths that provide autonomy over schedule and work methods.

Accommodation planning involves identifying workplace modifications you'll likely need throughout your career and developing strategies for accessing them. Research companies known for disability inclusion, prepare documentation that you can use across different positions, or develop networks with other autistic professionals who can share accommodation strategies.

Professional network development creates support systems and advancement opportunities that work with your social energy patterns. Build relationships through professional organizations related to your interests, connect with other neurodivergent professionals through online networks, or develop mentoring relationships that support your career growth.

Skill development strategies focus on building capabilities that enhance your natural strengths while addressing areas that might limit your professional options. Develop technical skills that complement your attention to detail, build communication abilities that work with your direct style, or learn management approaches that suit your systematic thinking.

Transition planning prepares you for career changes, promotions, or workplace modifications that might affect your accommodation needs. Document successful strategies from previous positions, maintain relationships with supportive supervisors or colleagues, or develop portable systems that you can implement in new work environments.

Jennifer's career planning illustrates long-term strategies. She identified that her pattern recognition abilities and attention to detail made her well-suited for compliance work, chose positions with companies known for supporting employee differences, built a network of neurodivergent professionals in her field, and developed portable accommodation strategies that she could implement in different work environments throughout her career progression.

Creating Sustainable Professional Success

Professional success as an autistic woman requires building career strategies that honor your neurological differences while allowing you to contribute your unique strengths effectively. This approach often leads to more satisfying and sustainable careers than attempting to conform to neurotypical professional expectations.

Your attention to detail, deep focus abilities, and systematic thinking create professional value that many employers seek but few understand how to support effectively. Learning to advocate for your needs while demonstrating your capabilities helps create work environments where you can excel authentically.

The accommodations you need aren't weaknesses to hide—they're supports that allow you to perform at your highest level. When you approach workplace modifications as productivity tools rather than disability accommodations, you often find that employers are willing to provide support that benefits your entire team.

Building a sustainable career often requires patience as you identify work environments, roles, and colleagues that appreciate your contributions while supporting your needs. Each positive professional experience provides learning that helps you make better career choices and advocate more effectively in future positions.

Chapter 11: Medical Self-Advocacy

- Healthcare Navigation

Healthcare interactions for autistic women often feel like exercises in frustration, miscommunication, and medical gaslighting. Your direct communication style might be misinterpreted as rudeness, your sensory needs dismissed as preferences, and your autism-related health concerns minimized or misunderstood. Effective medical self-advocacy requires specific strategies that help you access appropriate care while managing the sensory and social demands of healthcare environments.

Research by Dr. Melanie Yergeau shows that autistic women face significant barriers in healthcare settings, including longer wait times for appropriate diagnoses, higher rates of medical trauma, and frequent dismissal of their reported symptoms (37). Understanding these systemic challenges helps you prepare for healthcare encounters and develop advocacy strategies that improve your care outcomes.

Communicating Effectively with Healthcare Providers

Medical appointments require complex communication that balances providing necessary information with managing time constraints and social expectations. Your direct communication style can be an asset when channeled effectively in healthcare settings.

Preparation strategies help you organize information and communicate your needs clearly within appointment time limits. Create written lists of symptoms, concerns, and questions before appointments, research your conditions and treatment options to participate knowledgeably in medical discussions, gather relevant medical history and medication information, or prepare specific examples that illustrate your symptoms or concerns.

Communication framework development helps you present information in ways that healthcare providers can understand and act upon effectively. Lead with your most serious concerns to ensure they receive attention, provide specific examples and timelines for symptoms, explain how issues affect your daily functioning and quality of life, or use medical terminology when you know it to demonstrate your knowledge and engagement.

Advocacy scripts prepare you for common healthcare scenarios that might require self-advocacy. Develop responses for when providers dismiss your concerns, prepare explanations for why certain treatments might not work for you, create language for requesting accommodations during medical procedures, or practice expressing disagreement with treatment recommendations diplomatically.

Documentation strategies ensure you have records of medical interactions and can track patterns in your health concerns. Take notes during appointments or ask providers to document key points, request copies of all test results and medical records, maintain personal health journals that track symptoms and treatment responses, or use audio recording (with permission) if note-taking is difficult during appointments.

Follow-up protocols help you maintain continuity and ensure your healthcare needs receive appropriate attention. Confirm understanding of treatment plans before leaving appointments, ask for written instructions for complex treatment protocols, schedule follow-up appointments before leaving the office, or establish communication preferences for ongoing care coordination.

Lisa's communication approach demonstrates these strategies. She prepared detailed symptom timelines before appointments, created specific questions about treatment options, practiced explaining how her autism affected her medical experiences, and maintained comprehensive health records that helped providers understand patterns in her symptoms and treatment responses.

Advocating for Autism-Informed Healthcare

Many healthcare providers lack training in autism, particularly as it presents in women. Advocating for autism-informed care requires educating providers while ensuring your medical needs receive appropriate attention.

Provider education helps healthcare professionals understand how autism affects your medical experiences and care needs. Share information about autism in women if providers seem unfamiliar with current research, explain how sensory sensitivities affect medical procedures and environments, describe communication preferences that help you interact effectively with medical staff, or provide resources about autism-informed healthcare practices.

Sensory accommodation requests ensure medical environments support your comfort and cooperation during care. Ask for appointment times that avoid busy periods in medical offices, request examination rooms with adjustable lighting, explain your need for advance warning before physical examinations or procedures, or ask about alternative positioning or techniques that accommodate sensory sensitivities.

Communication accommodation strategies help you interact effectively with medical staff despite potential differences in communication styles. Request written instructions for complex medical procedures or medication regimens, ask for advance information about what to expect during appointments or procedures, explain your need for processing time before making medical decisions, or request that providers avoid sudden changes in conversation topics.

Treatment modification advocacy ensures medical recommendations account for your autistic traits and needs. Discuss how autism might affect your response to medications or treatments, explain executive function challenges that might affect treatment compliance, request modifications to standard treatment protocols when necessary, or advocate for autism-specific considerations in mental health treatments.

Specialist referral advocacy helps you access healthcare providers with autism expertise when needed. Request referrals to providers with autism training when appropriate, research specialists' experience with autistic adults before scheduling appointments, ask about providers' familiarity with autism in women specifically, or seek second opinions when you feel your autism-related needs aren't being addressed adequately.

Jennifer's advocacy process illustrates effective approaches. She created a one-page summary of how autism affected her healthcare needs, shared research articles about autism in women with providers who seemed unfamiliar with current understanding, requested specific accommodations like dimmed lighting and advance warning for physical examinations, and advocated for referrals to specialists with autism training when her general practitioners couldn't address autism-specific concerns.

Managing Medical Sensory Sensitivities

Healthcare environments often create intense sensory challenges through fluorescent lighting, medical equipment sounds, antiseptic smells, and unexpected physical contact. Developing strategies for managing these sensitivities improves your comfort and cooperation during medical care.

Environmental preparation helps you anticipate and manage sensory challenges in medical settings. Research medical offices online to understand their layouts and environments, call ahead to ask about lighting options and noise levels, request appointments during quieter times of day, or ask about private or less stimulating examination rooms.

Personal accommodation strategies provide tools for managing unavoidable sensory challenges during medical appointments. Bring noise-canceling headphones or earplugs for waiting areas, wear sunglasses if fluorescent lighting causes discomfort, carry comfort items or fidget tools for regulation during waiting periods, or use breathing techniques that help manage sensory overwhelm.

Communication about sensory needs helps medical staff understand and accommodate your requirements. Explain specific sensory sensitivities that affect your comfort during examinations, request advance warning before medical staff touch you or use medical equipment, ask for modifications to standard procedures when sensory issues make them intolerable, or provide information about sensory accommodations that have worked in previous medical encounters.

Procedure modification requests ensure medical treatments account for your sensory processing differences. Ask for step-by-step explanations of what providers will do during examinations, request breaks during lengthy procedures if you become overwhelmed, discuss alternative positioning or techniques that reduce sensory distress, or negotiate timing modifications that allow you to prepare for sensory-intensive procedures.

Recovery planning addresses the sensory aftermath of medical appointments and procedures. Schedule downtime after medical appointments to recover from sensory overload, plan quiet activities following procedures that might cause sensory overwhelm, arrange transportation that minimizes additional sensory stress after appointments, or prepare comfort measures for managing post-appointment sensory sensitivity.

Maria's sensory management shows comprehensive strategies. She researched medical offices before scheduling appointments, called ahead to request examination rooms with natural lighting when possible, brought noise-canceling headphones for waiting areas, explained her sensory sensitivities to medical staff at the beginning of appointments, and scheduled medical appointments during her peak energy periods to better cope with sensory challenges.

Addressing Co-Occurring Conditions Common in Autistic Women

Autistic women experience higher rates of certain medical and mental health conditions that require specialized understanding and treatment approaches. Advocating for appropriate care requires knowledge about these connections and persistence in finding providers who understand them.

Anxiety and depression occur at higher rates in autistic women, often stemming from years of masking, social challenges, and sensory overwhelm. Seek mental health providers who understand autism-related anxiety rather than treating it as a separate condition, advocate for treatment approaches that account for sensory sensitivities and executive function differences, or request therapy modalities that work with your communication style and processing patterns.

Gastrointestinal issues affect many autistic individuals and might require specialized medical attention. Research gastroenterologists who understand autism-gut connections, document food sensitivities and digestive patterns for medical providers, advocate for testing that considers autism-related GI problems, or seek providers who understand how sensory issues affect eating patterns and nutrition.

Sleep disorders commonly affect autistic women and might require autism-informed treatment approaches. Find sleep specialists who understand autism-related sleep challenges, document sleep patterns and environmental factors that affect your rest, advocate for sleep studies that accommodate sensory sensitivities, or request sleep hygiene recommendations that account for executive function and sensory differences.

Reproductive health concerns might require providers who understand how autism affects gynecological care and reproductive choices. Seek gynecologists who can accommodate sensory sensitivities during examinations, discuss how autism might affect pregnancy and parenting decisions, advocate for pain management approaches that account for sensory processing differences, or request autism-informed care during reproductive health procedures.

Autoimmune conditions occur at higher rates in autistic individuals and might require specialized medical attention. Research rheumatologists or immunologists who understand autism-autoimmune connections, document symptoms that might be related to both autism and autoimmune conditions, advocate for testing that considers these connections, or seek providers who understand how sensory issues might affect autoimmune symptom reporting.

Rachel's condition management demonstrates comprehensive approaches. She found a psychiatrist who specialized in autism and anxiety, worked with a gastroenterologist who understood autism-gut connections, connected with a gynecologist who accommodated her sensory needs during examinations, and maintained detailed health records that helped providers understand the connections between her various health concerns and her autism.

Finding Mental Health Providers Who Understand Autism

Mental health care for autistic women requires providers who understand how autism affects emotional processing, communication, and therapeutic relationships. Finding these specialists often requires persistence and specific search strategies.

Provider research strategies help you identify mental health professionals with autism expertise. Search for therapists who specifically mention autism in their practice descriptions, contact autism organizations for provider referrals, research therapists' training backgrounds and specializations, or ask potential providers directly about their experience working with autistic adults.

Screening questions help you assess providers' understanding and approach before committing to ongoing therapy. Ask about their training in autism and neurodiversity, inquire about their understanding of masking and autistic burnout, discuss their approach to therapy modifications for autistic clients, or ask how they accommodate sensory and communication differences in therapy sessions.

Therapy modification advocacy ensures mental health treatment works with your autistic traits rather than against them. Request therapy approaches that account for your communication style and processing patterns, ask for environmental modifications that support your sensory comfort during sessions, discuss how masking and social exhaustion affect your therapeutic goals, or advocate for treatment approaches that build on your autistic strengths.

Treatment goal alignment helps ensure therapy addresses your actual needs rather than attempting to make you more neurotypical. Focus on goals like stress management, self-advocacy skills, or life strategy development rather than social skills training designed to help you mask more effectively, discuss how autism affects your relationships and work life, or seek support for processing your diagnosis and identity development.

Ongoing advocacy maintains appropriate care as your needs change or if providers don't meet your expectations. Communicate when therapy approaches aren't working for you, request modifications to treatment plans that don't account for your autism, seek second opinions if you feel your autism-related needs aren't being addressed, or change providers if necessary to find someone who truly understands autistic experiences.

Sarah's provider search illustrates effective strategies. She researched therapists online and called several offices to ask specifically about autism experience, interviewed potential providers about their understanding of masking and autistic burnout, chose a therapist who had specialized training in autism and used neurodiversity-affirming approaches, and advocated for therapy modifications that accounted for her sensory needs and communication preferences.

Navigating Reproductive Health as an Autistic Woman

Reproductive healthcare presents unique challenges for autistic women, requiring providers who understand how sensory sensitivities, communication differences, and autism-related health concerns affect gynecological care and reproductive choices.

Gynecological care accommodations help make routine examinations and procedures more tolerable and effective. Find providers who can accommodate sensory sensitivities during examinations, request advance explanations of procedures to reduce anxiety and prepare mentally, ask for environmental modifications like dimmed lighting or reduced noise, or discuss positioning alternatives that increase your comfort during examinations.

Contraception considerations require providers who understand how autism might affect birth control choices and experiences. Discuss how sensory sensitivities might affect different contraceptive methods, consider how executive function differences might affect pill-taking consistency, explore options that minimize medical appointments and routine procedures, or find methods that account for sensory preferences and aversions.

Pregnancy planning involves considering how autism affects parenting decisions and pregnancy experiences. Discuss genetic counseling if you're concerned about autism inheritance, consider how pregnancy might affect your sensory sensitivities and medication needs, plan for pregnancy care that accommodates your communication and environmental preferences, or research obstetric providers who understand autism in women.

Fertility treatment considerations require providers who understand how autism affects treatment experiences and decision-making processes. Find fertility specialists who can accommodate sensory sensitivities during procedures, request detailed explanations of treatment protocols to help with planning and preparation, discuss how autism might affect your experience of fertility treatments, or advocate for treatment approaches that account for your communication and processing preferences.

Menopause planning involves preparing for hormonal changes that might interact with autism symptoms and needs. Research how hormonal changes might affect autism symptoms like sensory sensitivities and executive function, find healthcare providers who understand these connections, discuss hormone therapy options that account for autism-related factors, or plan for menopause management that supports your overall health and wellbeing.

Amanda's reproductive health advocacy shows comprehensive approaches. She found a gynecologist who specialized in women with disabilities, discussed her sensory needs before examinations and developed accommodation strategies, researched contraceptive options that aligned with her sensory preferences and executive function patterns, and planned ahead for pregnancy care that would accommodate her autism-related needs.

Building a Healthcare Team That Works

Effective healthcare for autistic women often requires coordination among multiple providers who understand autism and communicate effectively with each other about your needs and care.

Primary care coordination ensures your main healthcare provider understands your autism and can coordinate care appropriately. Find a primary care physician who has autism training or willingness to learn, provide comprehensive information about how autism affects your health and healthcare experiences, ensure your primary provider communicates effectively with specialists about your autism-related needs, or maintain organized medical records that help providers understand your health patterns and needs.

Specialist network development creates a team of healthcare providers who understand autism and can address your specific health concerns effectively. Research specialists who have autism training or experience, request referrals to providers who understand autism-related health concerns, maintain communication between specialists about your autism and its effects on treatment, or develop relationships with providers who can coordinate care effectively.

Emergency care planning prepares you for healthcare crises when you might not be able to advocate effectively for yourself. Create medical information summaries that explain your autism and accommodation needs, prepare emergency contact lists that include advocates who understand your needs, research emergency departments and urgent care centers that might be more autism-friendly, or develop crisis plans that address your autism-related needs during medical emergencies.

Medication management requires providers who understand how autism might affect medication responses and compliance. Find pharmacists who can accommodate your communication preferences and sensory needs, discuss with prescribers how autism might affect your medication experiences, maintain detailed records of medication responses and side effects, or develop systems that support medication compliance despite executive function challenges.

Health maintenance planning ensures you receive appropriate preventive care despite potential challenges with routine medical appointments. Schedule regular check-ups during times and with providers that work best for your needs, maintain organized records of health screenings and preventive care, advocate for modified screening procedures when standard protocols don't work for you, or develop systems that help you stay on top of routine healthcare needs.

Jennifer's team building demonstrates comprehensive approaches. She found a primary care physician who was willing to learn about autism and accommodate her needs, built relationships with specialists who had autism training or experience, created detailed medical summaries that she shared with all providers, developed emergency care plans that addressed her autism-related needs, and maintained organized health records that helped her coordinate care effectively across multiple providers.

The Foundation for Health and Advocacy

Effective medical self-advocacy as an autistic woman requires persistence, preparation, and the courage to educate providers while demanding appropriate care. Your health needs are legitimate, your sensory requirements deserve accommodation, and your autism-related concerns merit professional attention and expertise.

Building positive relationships with healthcare providers who understand autism often takes time and multiple attempts, but these connections become invaluable for maintaining your health and wellbeing throughout your life. Each successful healthcare interaction provides learning that helps you advocate more effectively in future medical encounters.

Your direct communication style and attention to detail can be significant assets in healthcare settings when you learn to channel them effectively. Providers often appreciate patients who come prepared with organized information and can communicate clearly about their symptoms and needs.

The healthcare system wasn't designed with autistic women in mind, but you can create positive healthcare experiences through strategic advocacy, provider education, and building relationships with professionals who appreciate and accommodate your differences while providing excellent medical care.

Chapter 12: Creating Your Support Network

- Building Comprehensive Life Support

Living authentically as an autistic woman requires a carefully constructed support network that understands your needs, appreciates your strengths, and provides assistance across the multiple domains where autism affects daily life. This network isn't built overnight—it develops gradually through intentional relationship-building, clear communication about your needs, and strategic connection with resources that truly understand and support neurodivergent experiences.

Dr. Ari Ne'eman's research on autistic community building emphasizes that effective support networks for autistic adults combine professional services, peer connections, and family relationships in ways that honor autonomy while providing necessary assistance (38). The key lies in creating support systems that empower rather than infantilize, accommodate rather than attempt to fix, and celebrate your authentic self while helping you navigate a neurotypical world.

Identifying Your Support Needs Across Life Domains

Creating an effective support network begins with honest assessment of where you need assistance, what types of support work best for you, and which life areas require different kinds of help at different times.

Daily living support might include assistance with executive function challenges, help managing overwhelming tasks, support for sensory regulation, or backup systems for times when autism burnout affects your functioning. These needs often fluctuate based on stress levels, life circumstances, and your overall energy and resources.

Professional support encompasses career guidance that understands autistic strengths and challenges, workplace accommodation advocacy, networking assistance that accounts for your social energy patterns, or career development that aligns with your neurological needs and interests rather than conventional career expectations.

Healthcare navigation requires advocates who understand autism in women, assistance with medical appointment preparation and follow-up, support for communicating with healthcare providers, or help coordinating care among multiple specialists who may not understand autism connections.

Social and emotional support involves relationships that appreciate your authentic self, understanding of your communication style and social energy patterns, assistance processing emotional experiences through your autistic lens, or connections with others who share similar experiences and challenges.

Crisis support includes people who understand your autism-related vulnerabilities, systems for managing overwhelming situations, assistance during burnout periods, or emergency contacts who can advocate for your needs when you can't advocate for yourself.

Lisa's needs assessment illustrates this process. She identified that she needed executive function support for managing household tasks during stressful periods, professional guidance for navigating workplace accommodations, healthcare advocacy for communicating with providers who didn't understand autism, social support from other autistic women who understood her experiences, and crisis support for managing sensory overload and burnout episodes.

Building Professional Support Teams

Professional support providers can offer specialized expertise and formal services that family and friends can't provide, but finding professionals who understand autism in women requires research, persistence, and clear communication about your needs.

Therapist selection should prioritize providers with autism expertise who use neurodiversity-affirming approaches. Look for therapists who understand masking, autistic burnout, and the specific challenges autistic women face, avoid providers who focus on making you more neurotypical rather than supporting your authentic self, or seek professionals who understand trauma-informed care for autistic individuals.

Life coaches and organizers can provide practical assistance with executive function challenges, daily life management, and goal achievement in ways that work with your autistic brain. Choose coaches who understand neurodivergent learning styles, seek providers who can help you build systems rather than forcing neurotypical approaches, or find organizers who appreciate your sensory needs and thinking patterns.

Medical advocates help you navigate healthcare systems and communicate effectively with providers who may not understand autism. Look for advocates with disability rights experience, seek individuals who understand autism in

146

women specifically, or find advocates who can accompany you to important medical appointments and help ensure your needs are understood and addressed.

Educational advocates support you in accessing appropriate accommodations in educational settings or help you advocate for neurodivergent children. Choose advocates with autism expertise and special education law knowledge, seek individuals who understand the challenges autistic women face in educational environments, or find advocates who can help you develop self-advocacy skills for future situations.

Career counselors who understand neurodivergent career development can help you find work that aligns with your strengths and accommodates your needs. Look for counselors who understand autistic career patterns and challenges, seek providers who can help you identify careers that leverage your strengths, or find counselors who understand workplace accommodation strategies and disclosure decisions.

Financial planners who understand disability-related financial planning can help you prepare for potential periods of reduced income due to burnout or discrimination, plan for accommodation-related expenses, or develop financial strategies that account for the unique career patterns many autistic women experience.

Jennifer's professional team building demonstrates strategic approaches. She found a therapist who specialized in autism and trauma, connected with a life coach who understood executive function differences, established a relationship with a disability rights advocate who could help with workplace issues, and worked with a career counselor who had experience supporting neurodivergent professionals in her field.

Creating Family Support Systems

Family support can be incredibly powerful when family members understand autism and learn to accommodate your needs, but building this understanding often requires ongoing education, clear communication, and patience as relatives adjust their expectations and behaviors.

Family education helps relatives understand how autism affects your daily life and what support you need from them. Share information about autism in women that counters stereotypes and misconceptions, explain your specific traits and how they affect your experiences, provide examples of helpful versus unhelpful responses to your needs, or recommend resources that help family members learn about supporting autistic adults.

Boundary establishment creates clear expectations about what you need from family relationships while respecting their limitations and boundaries. Communicate your sensory needs during family gatherings, explain your social energy patterns and how they affect family participation, establish protocols for family communication that work with your processing style, or set limits on family members' attempts to "fix" or change your autistic traits.

Accommodation negotiation helps family members understand specific modifications that make family interactions more successful for everyone. Request advance notice for family plans and gatherings, ask for environmental modifications during family events, explain your need for quiet spaces or breaks during family activities, or negotiate family traditions that accommodate your sensory and social needs.

Crisis support planning ensures family members understand how to help during difficult periods. Educate family about signs of autistic burnout or sensory overload, develop protocols for family assistance during overwhelming periods, establish emergency contact systems that work for your communication preferences, or create backup plans for family responsibilities when you can't fulfill usual roles.

Mutual support development creates family relationships that provide support to everyone rather than placing all accommodation burden on others. Identify ways your autistic traits benefit family functioning, offer your strengths to help with family challenges, develop reciprocal support systems that honor everyone's needs, or create family activities that work well for your neurological differences.

Maria's family system development shows effective strategies. She educated her family about autism in women through sharing articles and books, explained how her sensory sensitivities affected family gatherings and requested specific accommodations, established regular family communication about what was working and what needed adjustment, and developed ways to contribute her organizational skills to family planning and problem-solving.

Leveraging Online Communities Effectively

Online autistic communities provide access to understanding, information, and support that might not be available locally, but navigating these spaces effectively requires understanding their benefits and limitations while protecting your emotional wellbeing.

Community selection involves finding online spaces that align with your values and support your growth. Look for communities that emphasize neurodiversity and autism acceptance rather than cure-focused approaches, seek spaces that specifically support women and address their unique experiences, avoid communities that promote harmful stereotypes or self-hatred, or find groups that match your interests and life circumstances.

Participation strategies help you engage meaningfully while protecting your energy and emotional wellbeing. Start by observing community dynamics before actively participating, share your experiences in ways that feel comfortable and safe, offer support to others based on your capacity and expertise, or ask questions that help you learn and connect with others.

Information evaluation becomes crucial in online spaces where advice and information quality varies widely. Verify medical or legal advice with qualified professionals, distinguish between personal experiences and universal truths, critically evaluate information before implementing suggestions, or seek multiple perspectives on important decisions.

Boundary management protects you from online drama, toxic interactions, or overwhelming emotional content. Set limits on time spent in online communities, use privacy settings to control access to your personal information, avoid engaging in arguments or conflicts that drain your energy, or leave communities that become negative or harmful to your wellbeing.

Real-world connection helps you translate online relationships into practical support when possible and appropriate. Attend local meetups organized through online communities, develop deeper relationships with community members who live nearby, organize activities that bring online friends together in person, or maintain online relationships that provide support even without in-person contact.

Crisis support protocols ensure online communities can provide help during difficult periods while maintaining appropriate boundaries. Identify community members who understand crisis support and can provide assistance, establish communication methods for reaching out during overwhelming periods, develop safety plans that include online support resources, or maintain professional support alongside online community connections.

Rachel's online engagement illustrates balanced approaches. She joined several autism-focused Facebook groups and found one that particularly resonated with her experiences, participated regularly by sharing her experiences and supporting others, verified advice and information with her therapist and other professionals, established real-world friendships with several community members, and developed online support systems that helped during difficult periods while maintaining professional support relationships.

Connecting with Local Autism Organizations

Local autism organizations can provide in-person support, advocacy assistance, and connections to regional resources, but finding organizations that support autistic adults—particularly women—rather than focusing exclusively on children or family members requires research and evaluation.

Organization research helps you identify local groups that align with your needs and values. Look for organizations led by autistic individuals rather than only parents or professionals, seek groups that support autistic adults specifically rather than focusing only on children, evaluate organizations' approaches to ensure they emphasize acceptance rather than cure-focused messaging, or research their programs and services to determine relevance to your needs.

Program evaluation ensures activities and services actually benefit autistic adults rather than primarily serving other constituencies. Attend meetings or events to assess whether they provide meaningful support for your experiences, evaluate whether programming addresses real needs of autistic adults, assess whether the organization's leadership and decision-making includes autistic voices, or determine if services are accessible and accommodate sensory and communication differences.

Volunteer opportunities can provide ways to contribute your skills while building connections with the autism community. Offer your professional expertise to help with organizational challenges, contribute your special interests to program development or educational efforts, use your lived experience to help other autistic individuals, or provide support for advocacy efforts that benefit the broader autistic community.

Advocacy participation allows you to contribute to systemic change while building community connections. Join efforts to improve autism services and policies in your area, participate in disability rights advocacy that includes autism issues, support legislative efforts that benefit autistic adults, or contribute to public education efforts that increase autism understanding and acceptance.

Leadership development helps you build skills while creating positive change in autism community organizations. Seek training opportunities in disability rights advocacy, develop skills in nonprofit leadership and community organization, learn about autism policy and systems change, or build expertise in areas that benefit the broader autistic community.

Network building through organization involvement creates connections that extend beyond formal programming. Meet other autistic adults who share your interests and experiences, connect with families who understand and support autistic individuals, build relationships with professionals who work with the autism community, or develop connections with advocates and community leaders who can provide guidance and support.

Amy's organization involvement demonstrates comprehensive engagement. She researched local autism organizations and found one that was led by autistic adults and focused on acceptance rather than cure, attended meetings and events to assess whether they met her needs, volunteered her professional writing skills to help with newsletters and advocacy materials, participated in local advocacy efforts to improve autism services, and built lasting friendships with other autistic women through organization activities.

Developing Mentorship and Peer Support

Mentorship relationships—both being mentored and mentoring others—provide unique support that combines personal understanding with guidance and encouragement. These relationships often develop naturally through shared interests, professional connections, or community involvement.

Finding mentors involves identifying autistic women who have experiences or achievements you admire and developing relationships that provide guidance and support. Look for mentors through professional organizations in your field, connect with autistic women who have successfully navigated challenges you're facing, seek guidance from individuals who have built careers or lives that inspire you, or find mentors through autism community organizations and online spaces.

Mentorship relationship development requires clear communication about expectations, boundaries, and goals while allowing relationships to develop naturally. Communicate your goals and what you hope to learn from mentorship, establish boundaries around time and availability that work for both parties, express appreciation for guidance and support you receive, or maintain relationships that provide mutual benefit and connection rather than one-sided assistance.

Peer support creation involves building relationships with other autistic women who share similar experiences and can provide mutual understanding and assistance. Connect with women who are at similar life stages or facing comparable challenges, develop relationships that allow mutual support and encouragement, create informal support networks that provide regular connection and assistance, or participate in peer support groups that bring together women with shared experiences.

Mentoring others provides opportunities to contribute your knowledge and experience while building meaningful connections with other autistic women. Share your professional expertise with women entering your field, provide guidance about autism-related challenges you've successfully navigated, offer support for women who are newly diagnosed or struggling with similar issues, or contribute to formal mentorship programs through autism organizations or professional associations.

Skill sharing creates mutually beneficial relationships where you can learn from others while contributing your own expertise. Exchange knowledge about different professional fields or life experiences, share strategies for managing autism-related challenges, learn new skills from others while teaching your areas of expertise, or create informal learning partnerships that benefit everyone involved.

Community building through mentorship and peer support helps create networks that support multiple autistic women. Facilitate connections between autistic women who could support each other, organize gatherings or activities that bring together women with shared interests, create ongoing support groups that meet regularly, or contribute to building communities that provide sustained support over time.

Sarah's mentorship development illustrates these approaches. She connected with an autistic woman in her profession who became a valuable mentor, developed peer support relationships with several women through online autism communities, began mentoring newly diagnosed women who reached out for guidance, created a monthly virtual coffee meetup for autistic women in her area, and built lasting relationships that provided mutual support and encouragement.

Planning for Long-term Support and Aging

Creating support systems that can adapt and grow with you throughout your life requires thinking beyond current needs to consider how aging, life changes, and potential health issues might affect your support requirements.

Future needs assessment involves considering how your support needs might change as you age and face different life circumstances. Think about how autism-related challenges might change with aging, consider potential health issues that could affect your independence, plan for changes in your professional and family circumstances, or anticipate how your capacity for managing daily life might fluctuate over time.

Financial planning for support needs helps ensure you can access necessary assistance throughout your life. Plan for potential periods of reduced income due to burnout or discrimination, consider costs of professional support services you might need, research disability benefits and support programs you might be eligible for, or develop financial strategies that account for autism-related expenses and support needs.

Legal planning protects your autonomy while ensuring you have support for decision-making if needed. Create advance directives that reflect your values and preferences, consider power of attorney arrangements with people who understand your autism, research guardianship alternatives that preserve your autonomy, or develop legal documents that ensure your support needs are understood and met.

Housing considerations account for how your sensory and social needs might affect your living situation as you age. Consider housing options that provide community while accommodating your need for quiet and control over your environment, research accessible housing that accounts for potential mobility or health issues, plan for living arrangements that provide support without sacrificing independence, or explore intentional communities that include other neurodivergent individuals.

Healthcare planning ensures you'll have access to autism-informed medical care throughout your life. Maintain relationships with healthcare providers who understand autism in women, document your health history and accommodation needs for future providers, research healthcare systems and insurance options that provide appropriate coverage, or develop healthcare directives that ensure your autism-related needs are understood and respected.

Support system sustainability involves building networks that can continue providing assistance even as individual relationships change. Develop multiple sources of support rather than depending on single individuals, maintain connections with younger autistic women who might provide future support, contribute to autism community organizations that could provide assistance as you age, or build reciprocal support relationships that benefit everyone involved over time.

Amanda's long-term planning demonstrates comprehensive approaches. She worked with a financial planner who understood disability-related financial planning, created legal documents that protected her autonomy while ensuring support for decision-making, researched housing options that would accommodate her sensory needs as she aged, maintained relationships with autism-informed healthcare providers, and contributed to autism community organizations that could provide support throughout her life.

The Ongoing Journey of Support Network Development

Building a support network that truly understands and accommodates your autistic needs is an ongoing process that requires patience, persistence, and the courage to communicate your needs clearly while setting appropriate boundaries with the people who want to help you.

Your support network should empower your authentic self-expression rather than encouraging you to mask or conform to neurotypical expectations. The best support relationships celebrate your autistic traits while providing assistance with areas where you face genuine challenges or barriers.

Effective support networks often require you to educate others about autism and your specific needs, but this education investment pays dividends in relationships that truly understand and accommodate your neurological differences. Each person who learns to support you authentically becomes an advocate for broader autism acceptance and understanding.

The support you receive often becomes most meaningful when you can also contribute your strengths and expertise to help others. Mutual support relationships tend to be more sustainable and satisfying than one-sided assistance, creating communities that benefit everyone involved while building broader understanding and acceptance of neurodiversity.

Foundations for Lifelong Support

Creating a support network that sustains you through all of life's changes and challenges requires intentional planning, ongoing relationship maintenance, and the wisdom to seek help that empowers rather than diminishes your autonomy and authentic self-expression.

Your autism brings unique strengths that contribute to your support relationships and communities. The attention to detail, loyalty, and deep capacity for caring that characterize many autistic women often make you a valuable friend, colleague, and community member whose contributions strengthen the networks you're part of.

The support network you build becomes a model for other autistic women who may struggle to find understanding and accommodation in their own relationships and communities. Your success in creating authentic support demonstrates that autistic women can build rich, meaningful lives surrounded by people who appreciate and celebrate their neurodivergent identities.

The journey of building authentic support continues throughout your life, adapting to changing circumstances while maintaining the core principle that you deserve relationships and assistance that honor your authentic self while providing the understanding and accommodation that allow you to thrive as an autistic woman.

Key Principles for Lasting Support:

- Support networks should empower authentic self-expression rather than encouraging masking or conformity

- Professional support providers need autism expertise and neurodiversity-affirming approaches to be truly helpful

- Family support requires ongoing education and clear communication about your needs and boundaries

- Online communities provide valuable connection but require careful navigation and boundary management

- Local autism organizations can offer in-person support when they're led by autistic voices and focus on acceptance

- Mentorship and peer support create reciprocal relationships that benefit everyone involved

- Long-term planning ensures your support needs will be met throughout all life stages and circumstances

Appendix A: Assessment Tools and Checklists

Self-assessment tools provide starting points for understanding your autistic traits and patterns, but they're not substitutes for professional diagnosis. These checklists help you organize your observations and experiences before seeking professional evaluation or simply to better understand yourself. Each tool focuses on different aspects of the autistic experience and should be used thoughtfully rather than as definitive measures.

Use these assessments to identify patterns rather than to diagnose yourself. The goal is awareness and self-understanding that can guide your next steps, whether that's seeking professional evaluation, developing accommodation strategies, or simply gaining clarity about your experiences.

Female Autism Trait Checklist

This checklist addresses autism traits as they commonly appear in women and girls, accounting for masking behaviors and internalized presentations that traditional assessments often miss.

Social Communication and Interaction Patterns

Rate each item on a scale where: **Always** = occurs consistently across situations, **Often** = happens in most circumstances, **Sometimes** = appears in certain situations, **Rarely** = occurs infrequently, **Never** = doesn't apply to your experience.

- I feel like I'm acting or performing during social interactions rather than being naturally myself

- I study other people's behavior to learn appropriate social responses and copy what they do

- I have developed scripts or prepared responses for common social situations like small talk

- I prefer one-on-one conversations over group discussions because they feel more manageable

- I find it difficult to know when it's my turn to speak in conversations or group settings

- I take things literally and sometimes miss sarcasm, jokes, or implied meanings in conversations

- I feel exhausted after social events, even ones I enjoyed, and need time alone to recover

- I have intense, focused friendships rather than large groups of casual acquaintances

- I prefer friendships built around shared interests rather than general socializing

- I find workplace social dynamics like office politics confusing and draining to navigate

Sensory Processing Differences

- Certain sounds cause me physical discomfort or emotional distress, even when others don't notice them

- I'm sensitive to lighting and prefer specific types or levels of illumination for comfort

- Clothing textures, tags, or seams can be distracting or uncomfortable throughout the day

- I have strong preferences for specific foods based on texture, temperature, or other sensory qualities

- Crowded or busy environments quickly become overwhelming and make it hard to focus

- I seek out specific sensory experiences like particular fabrics, sounds, or movements for comfort

- I notice smells more intensely than others and some scents can trigger headaches or nausea

- I have difficulty filtering background noise and find it hard to focus in noisy environments

- Touch from others can feel uncomfortable or overwhelming, even when it's meant to be comforting

- I need to control my environment's temperature, lighting, or sound levels to feel comfortable

Restricted Interests and Repetitive Behaviors

- I have interests that others consider unusually intense or detailed for typical casual hobbies

- I enjoy researching topics thoroughly and becoming highly knowledgeable about specific subjects

- I prefer routines and feel unsettled when plans change unexpectedly or without advance notice

- I engage in repetitive movements or behaviors that help me think, focus, or feel calm

- I organize my belongings in specific ways and feel distressed when others move or disrupt them

- I have collections or hobbies that bring me deep satisfaction and occupy significant time

- I prefer doing familiar activities rather than trying new things that feel unpredictable

- I notice patterns and details that others miss in environments, objects, or information

- I have specific ways of doing routine tasks and feel frustrated when I can't follow them

- I find comfort in familiar objects, places, or activities during stressful periods

Executive Function and Daily Life Management

- I struggle with tasks that have multiple steps or require planning several things simultaneously

- Time management feels challenging and I often underestimate or overestimate how long tasks will take

- I have difficulty starting tasks even when I know exactly what needs to be done

- Transitions between activities or locations feel difficult and require mental preparation

- I work better with clear structures, deadlines, and detailed instructions rather than open-ended tasks

- I become overwhelmed when facing too many choices or decisions at once

164

- I have difficulty prioritizing tasks when everything feels equally important or urgent

- Organization systems that work for others don't match how my brain naturally processes information

- I procrastinate on important tasks but can focus intensely on things that interest me

- I need visual reminders, lists, or external structures to maintain organization and complete tasks

Emotional Regulation and Self-Awareness

- I have difficulty identifying and naming my emotions, especially in the moment they occur

- I experience emotions very intensely, and small frustrations can feel overwhelming

- I have meltdowns or shutdowns when I become too overwhelmed to cope with demands

- I mask my real emotions and reactions to appear more socially acceptable to others

- I find it hard to recognize when I'm becoming overwhelmed until I reach a breaking point

- I have difficulty advocating for my needs because I struggle to identify what I need

- I feel different from other people in ways I can't easily explain or articulate

- I have been told I'm "too sensitive" or that I "overreact" to situations others handle easily

- I prefer to process emotional experiences privately rather than discussing them immediately

- I have strong emotional reactions to things like injustice, changes in routine, or sensory overwhelm

Childhood and Developmental History

- I was described as a "good girl," "mature for my age," or "in my own world" during childhood

- I preferred reading, creative activities, or solitary play over typical childhood social games

- I had intense interests in specific topics that seemed unusual for my age or gender

- I struggled with changes in routine, new environments, or unexpected social demands as a child

- I was extremely rule-following and became distressed when others broke rules or expectations

- I had difficulty making friends or maintaining typical childhood social relationships

- I was often described as shy, sensitive, or requiring special handling in social situations

- I developed elaborate fantasy worlds or engaged in detailed imaginative play for hours

- I had strong reactions to sensory experiences like clothing textures, food textures, or loud sounds

- I learned social behaviors by watching and copying others rather than understanding them naturally

Scoring and Interpretation Guide

Count how many items you rated as "Always" or "Often" across all categories. Higher numbers of frequent experiences suggest stronger alignment with autistic traits, but this checklist doesn't provide a diagnostic score or threshold.

Over 40 items rated "Always" or "Often" suggests significant alignment with autistic traits and may warrant professional evaluation.

Between 25-40 items indicates moderate alignment that might benefit from further exploration and self-understanding.

Under 25 items suggests fewer autistic traits, though this doesn't rule out autism, particularly if your experiences have been masked or internalized.

Focus on patterns rather than total numbers. Strong clustering in specific areas like sensory processing or social communication might be more significant than scattered items across categories.

Sensory Profile Assessment

Understanding your sensory processing patterns helps you identify environmental modifications and self-regulation strategies that support your daily functioning and wellbeing.

Auditory Processing Evaluation

For each sound or acoustic situation, rate your typical response using: **Seek** = actively enjoy or pursue this experience, **Tolerate** = can handle without significant distress, **Avoid** = actively try to prevent or minimize exposure, **Overwhelm** = causes significant distress or shutdown.

- Background conversations in restaurants or busy environments

- Sudden loud noises like alarms, sirens, or doors slamming

- Repetitive sounds like ticking clocks, dripping faucets, or humming electronics

- Music with heavy bass, complex rhythms, or multiple instruments playing simultaneously

- Vacuum cleaners, blenders, hair dryers, or other household appliances

- Crowds of people talking, laughing, or making noise in public spaces

- Telephone rings, notification sounds, or electronic beeps and alerts

- Construction noise, traffic sounds, or urban environmental noise

- Children crying, screaming, or making high-pitched vocalizations

- Specific music, nature sounds, or audio that you find particularly calming or focusing

Visual Processing Assessment

- Fluorescent lighting in offices, stores, or public buildings

- Bright sunlight or high-contrast lighting situations

- Flickering lights, strobe effects, or rapidly changing visual displays

- Cluttered visual environments with many objects, patterns, or competing elements

- Certain colors, patterns, or visual textures that feel uncomfortable to look at

- Moving objects like ceiling fans, spinning wheels, or flowing water

- Computer screens, television displays, or digital devices for extended periods

- Peripheral movement or activity while trying to focus on central tasks

- Specific visual patterns, colors, or arrangements that feel particularly calming

- Natural lighting, specific color temperatures, or preferred visual environments

Tactile Processing Patterns

- Light touch from other people, including hugs, handshakes, or casual contact

- Specific clothing textures like wool, synthetic fabrics, or rough materials

- Temperature variations including very hot or cold objects, weather, or environments

- Sticky, wet, or messy textures from foods, art supplies, or environmental contact

- Hair washing, face washing, or other personal care activities involving touch

- Deep pressure touch like tight hugs, weighted blankets, or firm massage

- Smooth textures like silk, satin, or polished surfaces that feel particularly pleasant

- Rough textures like sandpaper, concrete, or coarse fabrics

- Unexpected touch from others or contact that occurs without warning

- Self-stimulating touch behaviors like fabric rubbing, hair twisting, or skin picking

Olfactory and Gustatory Sensitivities

- Strong perfumes, colognes, or artificial fragrances in products or environments

- Food smells, cooking odors, or restaurant environments with complex scent combinations

- Chemical smells from cleaning products, gasoline, or industrial environments

- Body odors, including your own or others' natural scents

- Specific food textures that affect your eating preferences and meal planning

- Temperature preferences in foods and beverages that affect your comfort

- Spicy, sour, bitter, or intensely flavored foods and seasonings

- Mixed textures in foods like casseroles, smoothies, or combination dishes

- Natural scents like flowers, essential oils, or outdoor environments that feel calming

- Specific taste combinations or food preparations that you particularly enjoy or crave

Proprioceptive and Vestibular Responses

- Activities involving balance like climbing stairs, walking on uneven surfaces, or riding elevators

- Movement activities like swinging, spinning, or riding in vehicles

- Deep pressure activities like heavy lifting, tight spaces, or compression

- Spatial awareness challenges like bumping into objects or misjudging distances

- Activities requiring fine motor control like writing, typing, or detailed manipulation

- Gross motor activities like sports, dancing, or coordinated physical movement

- Position changes like standing up quickly, bending over, or changing orientation

- Activities that provide strong proprioceptive input like jumping, pushing, or pulling

- Stillness or lack of movement that feels uncomfortable or makes focus difficult
- Specific movements or positions that help you feel grounded and regulated

Interoceptive Awareness

- Recognizing hunger signals and knowing when you need to eat
- Identifying thirst and remembering to drink fluids throughout the day
- Noticing when you need to use the bathroom before it becomes urgent
- Recognizing fatigue and understanding when you need rest or sleep
- Identifying emotional states and connecting them to physical sensations
- Noticing pain, discomfort, or illness symptoms in your body
- Recognizing when you're becoming overwhelmed before reaching crisis points
- Understanding your body's temperature regulation needs
- Identifying stress or anxiety through physical sensations
- Connecting environmental factors to changes in how your body feels

Environmental Processing Evaluation

Rate your comfort and functioning in different environmental contexts:

- Open office spaces with multiple people, conversations, and activities

- Crowded public spaces like malls, airports, or busy streets

- Quiet, controlled environments like libraries, empty offices, or your bedroom

- Natural outdoor environments like parks, forests, or beaches

- Social gatherings with background music, conversation, and multiple sensory inputs

- Medical environments with bright lights, equipment sounds, and clinical smells

- Restaurants with background noise, food smells, and social expectations

- Retail environments with fluorescent lighting, music, and visual stimulation

- Transportation environments like buses, planes, or crowded subway systems

- Home environments that you can control and modify to meet your preferences

Daily Sensory Pattern Tracking

Monitor your sensory experiences for one week, noting:

1. Times of day when you feel most/least comfortable sensorily

2. Environmental factors that consistently improve or worsen your functioning

3. Sensory experiences you actively seek for regulation or comfort

4. Situations that reliably trigger sensory overwhelm or shutdown

5. Accommodations or modifications that significantly improve your comfort

6. Patterns between sensory experiences and your energy, mood, or productivity

7. Seasonal or weather-related changes in your sensory sensitivity

8. Medications, foods, or other factors that affect your sensory processing

9. Social or emotional stressors that change your sensory tolerance

10. Recovery strategies that help you return to baseline after sensory overload

Masking Inventory

This assessment helps you identify masking behaviors you might engage in unconsciously and understand their impact on your energy and authenticity.

Social Masking Behaviors

Rate how often you engage in each behavior: **Always** = in every social situation, **Often** = in most social contexts, **Sometimes** = in specific situations, **Rarely** = only occasionally, **Never** = doesn't apply to you.

- I rehearse conversations in my head before social interactions

- I study other people's facial expressions and body language to copy appropriate responses

- I force myself to make eye contact even when it feels uncomfortable or draining

- I suppress my natural movements, fidgeting, or stimming behaviors in social situations

- I pretend to be interested in topics that don't actually engage me to fit in socially

- I modify my voice tone, volume, or speech patterns to sound more "normal"

- I agree with opinions I don't share to avoid conflict or standing out

- I prepare standard responses for common social questions like "How was your weekend?"

- I monitor my facial expressions to ensure they match what others expect

- I suppress my enthusiasm about special interests to avoid seeming "weird" or "obsessive"

Professional Masking Patterns

- I attend workplace social events despite preferring to skip them

- I participate in small talk and casual conversation even when it feels meaningless

- I volunteer for projects or responsibilities to prove I'm a team player

- I hide my need for accommodations like noise-canceling headphones or specific lighting

- I pretend that interruptions and multitasking don't affect my productivity

- I suppress visible signs of stress or overwhelm during work hours

- I mimic colleagues' communication styles rather than using my natural approach

- I attend meetings without requesting accommodations that would help me participate effectively

- I avoid requesting deadline extensions or task modifications even when I need them

- I perform enthusiasm about workplace culture or values that don't align with my own

Emotional Masking Strategies

- I smile and appear cheerful when I'm actually feeling overwhelmed or distressed

- I suppress meltdowns or shutdowns in public and wait until I'm alone to decompress

- I hide my emotional reactions to sensory overwhelm, social stress, or unexpected changes

- I pretend that criticism or feedback doesn't affect me as strongly as it actually does

176

- I minimize my emotional needs in relationships to avoid seeming "high-maintenance"

- I suppress strong positive emotions like excitement to avoid seeming "too much"

- I act calm and composed during situations that actually feel chaotic or overwhelming

- I hide my emotional processing time and pretend to respond immediately to complex situations

- I suppress my natural emotional intensity to match others' more moderate responses

- I pretend that social rejection or exclusion doesn't hurt as much as it actually does

Sensory Masking Efforts

- I endure uncomfortable sensory environments without requesting modifications

- I suppress visible reactions to sounds, lights, or textures that bother me

- I participate in activities despite sensory discomfort to avoid seeming difficult

- I wear clothing that's uncomfortable but socially appropriate rather than requesting alternatives

- I attend events in overwhelming environments without bringing sensory tools that would help

- I suppress stimming or self-regulation behaviors that would help me cope with sensory input

- I pretend that noisy or chaotic environments don't affect my ability to focus or function

- I endure physical discomfort from lighting, temperature, or acoustic conditions without complaining

- I participate in sensory-intensive activities like concerts or crowded events despite personal discomfort

- I avoid requesting environmental accommodations that would significantly improve my comfort

Communication Masking Techniques

- I use indirect communication instead of stating my needs or preferences directly

- I suppress my natural tendency to be precise or detailed in my communication

- I add unnecessary social pleasantries to make my communication seem more typical

- I pretend to understand social cues or implications that are actually unclear to me

- I modify my natural speaking rhythm, volume, or tone to sound more socially acceptable

- I suppress my tendency to ask clarifying questions about ambiguous instructions or expectations

- I pretend that sarcasm, jokes, or implied meanings are clear when they're actually confusing

- I use humor or deflection to avoid direct conversations about my needs or feelings

- I suppress my natural tendency to focus intensely on topics that interest me during conversations

- I modify my vocabulary or communication style to match what I think others expect

Identity Masking Patterns

- I hide my autism diagnosis or self-understanding from most people in my life

- I suppress interests, hobbies, or preferences that might seem unusual or intense

- I pretend to enjoy activities or experiences that don't actually bring me satisfaction

- I modify my appearance, behavior, or lifestyle to appear more neurotypical

- I suppress aspects of my personality that feel authentic but might be seen as different

- I pretend that my need for routine, structure, or predictability is less important than it is

- I hide my executive function challenges and struggle privately rather than requesting help

- I suppress my natural learning style and force myself to adapt to conventional approaches

- I pretend that my sensory preferences are casual choices rather than genuine needs

- I mask my autism-related strengths to avoid drawing attention to my differences

Physical and Energy Impact Assessment

Rate how masking affects your physical and emotional wellbeing:

- Chronic fatigue or exhaustion that doesn't improve with rest

- Headaches, muscle tension, or physical stress symptoms after social situations

- Difficulty sleeping or relaxing after periods of intensive masking

- Anxiety, depression, or emotional overwhelm related to maintaining your masked persona

- Loss of connection to your authentic self, interests, or preferences

- Difficulty identifying your genuine needs, feelings, or desires

- Resentment or frustration about needing to hide aspects of yourself

- Fear of being discovered or having your mask slip in social situations

- Confusion about your identity when you're constantly adapting to others' expectations

- Physical symptoms like digestive issues, immune problems, or chronic pain that might relate to stress

Masking Reduction Strategies

Identify areas where you might begin reducing masking safely:

1. **Low-risk environments** where authentic expression feels safer

2. **Trusted relationships** where you can practice being more genuine

3. **Professional accommodations** you could request without full disclosure

4. **Social situations** you could modify or avoid to reduce masking demands

5. **Communication changes** that would feel more authentic while remaining appropriate

6. **Environmental modifications** that would reduce your need to mask sensory responses

7. **Boundary setting** that protects your energy for situations that truly require masking

8. **Recovery strategies** that help you decompress after necessary masking periods

9. **Self-advocacy skills** that allow you to request accommodations confidently

10. **Support systems** that understand and appreciate your authentic self

Executive Function Evaluation

This assessment helps you identify specific executive function patterns and challenges so you can develop targeted strategies and accommodations.

Task Initiation and Planning Assessment

Rate your typical experience with each area: **Strength** = consistently easy for you, **Manageable** = you can do this with effort, **Challenging** = requires significant strategies or support, **Very Difficult** = major obstacle in daily life.

- Starting tasks even when you know exactly what needs to be done

- Breaking large projects into smaller, manageable steps

- Estimating how long tasks will take to complete accurately

- Planning the sequence of steps needed to complete complex activities

- Beginning work on projects that don't have immediate deadlines

- Initiating routine tasks like household chores or personal care without external prompts

- Starting creative or open-ended projects that don't have clear structure

- Beginning tasks that require multiple materials, tools, or preparation steps

- Initiating social contact or communication when you need to reach out to others

- Starting tasks that involve potential failure, criticism, or judgment from others

Working Memory and Attention Management

- Holding multiple pieces of information in mind while completing complex tasks

- Following multi-step instructions without writing them down or asking for repetition

- Maintaining focus on tasks when there are distractions in your environment

- Switching between different tasks or activities without losing track of where you left off

- Maintaining awareness of time passage while engaged in focused activities

- Tracking multiple ongoing projects or responsibilities simultaneously

- Maintaining attention during long meetings, lectures, or instructional periods

- Following conversations that involve multiple topics or participants

- Maintaining focus on boring or routine tasks that don't naturally engage your interest

- Managing attention when your hyperfocus shifts to topics that aren't currently priorities

Organization and Time Management

- Maintaining organized physical spaces like your desk, bedroom, or work area

- Keeping track of important documents, keys, and everyday items

- Managing calendar appointments and showing up on time for scheduled activities

- Prioritizing tasks when multiple things feel equally important or urgent

- Maintaining organizational systems consistently over time

- Managing your daily schedule to include both planned activities and unexpected demands

- Organizing digital files, emails, and electronic information in accessible ways

- Managing seasonal tasks like holiday planning, tax preparation, or annual appointments

- Coordinating complex schedules that involve multiple people or activities

- Maintaining household management tasks like bill paying, cleaning schedules, or maintenance

Cognitive Flexibility and Adaptation

- Adapting to unexpected changes in plans, schedules, or routines

- Switching strategies when your initial approach to a problem isn't working

- Handling interruptions during focused work without losing productivity or becoming frustrated

- Adapting your communication style for different audiences or social contexts

- Managing multiple competing priorities when they conflict with each other

- Adjusting expectations when situations change or new information becomes available

- Handling criticism or feedback that requires changing your approach to tasks or projects

- Adapting to new work environments, living situations, or social expectations

- Managing uncertainty about outcomes, timelines, or other people's decisions

- Adjusting routines when life circumstances change your usual patterns

Emotional Regulation and Self-Monitoring

- Recognizing when you're becoming overwhelmed before reaching crisis points

- Managing frustration when tasks take longer than expected or don't go as planned

- Maintaining motivation for long-term projects that don't provide immediate satisfaction

- Regulating your emotional responses during stressful or demanding situations

- Monitoring your energy levels and adjusting your commitments accordingly

- Managing perfectionism or all-or-nothing thinking that interferes with task completion

- Recognizing when you need breaks, help, or accommodations during demanding periods

- Managing anxiety or avoidance that prevents you from starting or completing important tasks

- Maintaining emotional equilibrium during periods of high demand or stress

- Recognizing and addressing procrastination patterns before they become problematic

Decision-Making and Problem-Solving

- Making decisions when facing multiple options that all seem equally valid or appealing

- Solving problems that require creative or unconventional approaches

- Making quick decisions under pressure without extensive analysis or preparation time

- Solving interpersonal problems that involve understanding others' perspectives or motivations

- Making decisions about priorities when resources like time, energy, or money are limited

- Problem-solving in situations that don't have clear rules, guidelines, or precedents

- Making decisions that involve risk, uncertainty, or potential negative consequences

- Solving problems that require coordinating with other people or getting consensus

- Making everyday decisions without excessive analysis or seeking input from others

- Problem-solving when your usual strategies or approaches aren't applicable

Daily Life Management Patterns

- Maintaining routines for personal care, nutrition, and health management

- Managing household responsibilities like cleaning, organization, and maintenance

- Coordinating transportation, appointments, and logistical requirements

- Managing financial responsibilities like budgeting, bill paying, and financial planning

- Maintaining social relationships and communication with family, friends, and colleagues

- Managing work responsibilities, deadlines, and professional development

- Coordinating childcare, pet care, or other dependent care responsibilities

- Managing seasonal or periodic tasks that don't occur on regular schedules

- Maintaining balance between work, personal, and family responsibilities

- Managing crisis situations or unexpected demands on your time and energy

Accommodation and Strategy Effectiveness

Evaluate which supports have helped you manage executive function challenges:

- **External structure** like calendars, reminders, or scheduling systems

- **Environmental modifications** that reduce distractions or support focus

- **Task breakdown** systems that make large projects more manageable

- **Deadline management** strategies that help you meet time commitments

- **Energy management** approaches that align tasks with your optimal functioning periods

- **Technology tools** that support organization, time management, or task completion

- **Support from others** who help with planning, accountability, or task completion

- **Routine development** that automates decision-making and reduces cognitive load

- **Priority clarification** systems that help you identify what's most important

- **Stress management** techniques that maintain your executive function during challenging periods

Pattern Recognition and Future Planning

Use your assessment results to identify:

1. **Consistent strengths** you can build upon and leverage for success

2. **Reliable challenges** that benefit from specific accommodations or strategies

3. **Situational factors** that improve or worsen your executive functioning

4. **Time patterns** when your executive function is strongest or most challenged

5. **Environmental factors** that support or hinder your cognitive organization

6. **Stress impacts** on your ability to plan, organize, and execute tasks

7. **Support needs** that would most significantly improve your daily functioning

8. **Accommodation priorities** that would provide the greatest benefit with reasonable effort

9. **Crisis prevention** strategies that help you avoid executive function breakdowns

10. **Long-term development** goals for building sustainable executive function support

Appendix B: Resource Directory

Finding qualified providers and reliable resources requires careful research, especially given the limited number of professionals who truly understand autism in women. This directory provides starting points for your search, but always verify current information and evaluate whether specific providers or resources meet your individual needs.

Diagnostic Providers by Region

Northeast Region

Massachusetts: Massachusetts General Hospital Autism Program in Boston provides adult autism evaluations with experience in female presentations. Harvard Medical School affiliates often have autism specialists, though wait times can be extensive. Contact autism organizations in the Boston area for current provider recommendations.

New York: Mount Sinai Hospital's Seaver Autism Center in New York City offers adult evaluations, though their focus is primarily research-oriented. Weill Cornell Medicine has providers experienced in adult autism assessment. Private practice psychologists in the New York metropolitan area often have shorter wait times than hospital systems.

Pennsylvania: University of Pennsylvania's autism research programs sometimes offer evaluations, particularly for research participants. Private practices in Philadelphia and Pittsburgh may provide more accessible assessment options.

Connecticut: Yale Child Study Center occasionally evaluates adults, particularly those participating in research studies. Connecticut's autism organizations can provide referrals to qualified private practitioners.

Southeast Region

Florida: University of Miami's autism research programs offer some adult evaluations. Florida Institute of Technology has autism specialists who work with adults. The large autism community in South Florida has created a network of private practitioners with experience in adult diagnosis.

North Carolina: University of North Carolina's autism research center provides some adult evaluations, particularly for research participants. Duke University's autism programs occasionally evaluate adults.

Georgia: Emory University's autism research programs offer limited adult evaluations. Marcus Autism Center in Atlanta focuses primarily on children but maintains referral networks for adults.

Virginia: Virginia Commonwealth University has autism specialists who work with adults. Northern Virginia's proximity to autism research centers provides access to qualified private practitioners.

Midwest Region

Illinois: University of Chicago's autism research programs offer some adult evaluations. Northwestern University has autism specialists experienced in adult assessment. The Chicago area has numerous private practitioners with autism expertise.

Michigan: University of Michigan's autism research center provides adult evaluations, particularly for research participants. Henry Ford Health System has autism specialists who work with adults.

Ohio: Cincinnati Children's Hospital occasionally evaluates adults transitioning from pediatric care. Ohio State University's autism programs have some adult-focused services.

Minnesota: University of Minnesota's autism research programs offer limited adult evaluations. Minneapolis-St. Paul area has private practitioners with autism specialization.

West Coast Region

California: UCLA's autism research center provides some adult evaluations, particularly for research studies. Stanford University's autism programs occasionally evaluate adults. University of California San Francisco has autism specialists with adult experience. The large autism community in California has created numerous private practice options.

Washington: University of Washington's autism research center offers adult evaluations, particularly for research participants. Seattle Children's Hospital occasionally evaluates adults transitioning from pediatric services.

Oregon: Oregon Health & Science University has autism specialists who work with adults. Portland's autism community provides referral networks for qualified practitioners.

Mountain and Plains Region

Colorado: University of Colorado's autism research programs offer some adult evaluations. Denver area private practitioners with autism specialization are available through autism organization referrals.

Texas: University of Texas Southwestern has autism specialists with adult experience. Baylor College of Medicine's autism programs occasionally evaluate adults. Houston and Dallas areas have private practitioners with autism expertise.

Arizona: Southwest Autism Research & Resource Center in Phoenix provides adult evaluations. Arizona State University's autism research programs offer limited adult assessment services.

Provider Selection Criteria

When evaluating potential diagnostic providers, ask these specific questions:

1. How many adult women have you diagnosed with autism in the past year?

2. Are you familiar with masking and camouflaging behaviors in women?

3. What assessment tools do you use specifically for adult women?

4. How do you account for female autism presentations that differ from traditional criteria?

5. What is your understanding of autism as a neurological difference versus a disorder?

6. How long is your assessment process and what does it include?

7. Do you provide written reports that can be used for accommodation requests?

8. What are your fees and do you accept insurance or offer payment plans?

9. How long is your current wait list for new adult evaluations?

10. Can you provide references from other autistic women you've diagnosed?

Recommended Books and Resources

Autism Understanding and Self-Discovery

Unmasking Autism by Devon Price provides excellent coverage of masking behaviors and late diagnosis experiences. Price's research-based approach combined with lived experience offers practical guidance for understanding autism in adults.

Women and Girls with Autism Spectrum Disorder by Sarah Hendrickx addresses the unique presentations and challenges faced by autistic females across the lifespan. This resource is particularly valuable for understanding how autism manifests differently in women.

Neurotribes by Steve Silberman offers historical context about autism research and the neurodiversity movement. This book helps readers understand how autism has been misunderstood and provides hope for future acceptance.

The Autistic Brain by Temple Grandin combines personal experience with scientific research to explain autism from both neurological and lived experience perspectives.

Professional and Workplace Resources

Asperger's on the Job by Rudy Simone provides practical strategies for workplace success, including disclosure decisions and accommodation requests.

The Complete Guide to Asperger's Syndrome by Tony Attwood offers detailed information about autism traits and strategies, though it uses older terminology.

Relationships and Social Connection

The Journal of Best Practices by David Finch provides insight into marriage and relationships when one partner is autistic, offering both humor and practical guidance.

Aspergirls by Rudy Simone focuses specifically on women and girls with autism, addressing relationships, careers, and daily life challenges.

Parenting Resources

Parenting Without Panic by Lynne Soraya offers guidance for autistic parents raising children, including strategies for managing sensory overwhelm and executive function challenges.

The Reason I Jump by Naoki Higashida provides insight into the autistic experience that can help autistic parents understand their children's perspectives.

Mental Health and Self-Care

The Autistic Survival Guide to Therapy by Kieran Rose offers guidance for finding appropriate mental health support and advocating for autism-informed therapy.

Autism and Masking by Kieran Rose addresses the mental health impacts of masking and strategies for authentic living.

Online Resources and Websites

The Autism Women's Network provides resources specifically for autistic women and girls, including support groups, advocacy information, and community connections.

Thinking Person's Guide to Autism offers evidence-based information about autism from autistic authors, parents, and professionals who support neurodiversity approaches.

The Autistic Self Advocacy Network provides advocacy resources, policy information, and community connections led by autistic individuals.

Neurodivergent Insights offers practical resources for understanding and supporting neurodivergent individuals in various life contexts.

Research and Academic Resources

PubMed database allows you to search for current autism research, particularly studies focusing on autism in women and girls.

Autism Research journal publishes current research about autism across the lifespan, including studies relevant to late diagnosis and female presentations.

Journal of Autism and Developmental Disorders provides academic research about autism that can inform your understanding of current scientific knowledge.

Apps and Technology Tools

Communication and Social Support

Marco Polo allows asynchronous video communication that works well for autistic communication patterns. You can send video messages when you have energy and respond when convenient.

Discord provides text and voice chat options that allow you to connect with autism communities and support groups online.

WhatsApp offers text messaging with international capabilities for connecting with autism communities worldwide.

Zoom or Google Meet facilitate virtual support group meetings and therapy sessions from your own environment.

Organization and Executive Function

Todoist provides task management with natural language processing that makes it easy to add tasks and organize projects without complex setup.

Forest helps with focus by gamifying distraction-free work periods using visual tree-growing metaphors.

RescueTime tracks how you spend time on digital devices, helping you understand your productivity patterns and energy cycles.

Google Calendar integrates across devices and allows detailed scheduling with location reminders and notification customization.

Notion combines note-taking, task management, and project organization in customizable formats that work well for autistic thinking patterns.

Sensory Management

Noisli provides customizable background sounds for focus and relaxation, including nature sounds and white noise options.

Twilight adjusts your device's screen color temperature to reduce blue light exposure that can affect sleep and sensory comfort.

Headspace offers guided meditation and mindfulness exercises that can help with emotional regulation and stress management.

Calm provides sleep stories, meditation, and relaxation resources that support sensory regulation and stress reduction.

Time and Schedule Management

TimeTree allows shared calendar management for families and support teams while maintaining individual privacy controls.

Due provides persistent reminders for important tasks and appointments until you mark them complete.

Hours tracks time spent on different activities, helping you understand your energy patterns and optimize your schedule.

Be Focused uses the Pomodoro Technique to structure work periods with built-in breaks that support attention management and prevent hyperfocus exhaustion.

Financial Management

Mint tracks expenses and budgets automatically, reducing the executive function demands of financial management.

YNAB (You Need A Budget) provides structured budgeting approaches that work well for systematic thinking patterns.

PocketGuard helps prevent overspending by tracking available funds in real-time.

Health and Self-Care Tracking

MyFitnessPal tracks nutrition and eating patterns, which can be helpful for identifying food sensitivities and maintaining consistent nutrition.

Sleep Cycle monitors sleep patterns and can help identify factors that affect your rest quality.

Mood Meter helps with emotional recognition and regulation by providing frameworks for identifying and naming feelings.

Daylio offers simple mood tracking with customizable factors that help you identify patterns in your emotional experiences.

Support Organizations and Communities

National Organizations

Autistic Self Advocacy Network (ASAN) provides policy advocacy, resources, and community connections led entirely by autistic individuals. Their approach emphasizes neurodiversity and civil rights rather than cure-focused messaging.

Autism Women's Network offers support specifically for autistic women and girls, including online support groups, resources, and advocacy efforts that address the unique challenges faced by females on the spectrum.

Autism Society of America provides local chapter connections, resource directories, and advocacy support, though their approach varies by local chapter and some focus more on families than autistic adults.

Online Community Platforms

Facebook groups for autistic women provide peer support and information sharing, but quality varies significantly between groups. Look for groups with clear community guidelines and moderation policies.

Reddit communities like r/aspergirls and r/autism offer discussion forums and support, though anonymity allows both helpful and harmful interactions.

Twitter hashtags like #ActuallyAutistic connect autistic voices and provide access to autism advocacy discussions and resource sharing.

Professional Support Networks

International Association of Autism Professionals includes providers who work specifically with autistic individuals, though membership doesn't guarantee autism expertise.

Association for Applied and Therapeutic Humor offers resources for therapists and counselors, including some who specialize in neurodivergent clients.

Local Community Building

Meetup.com often hosts autism support groups and social gatherings in urban areas, though quality and approach vary significantly.

University disability services offices sometimes host adult autism support groups or can provide referrals to local resources.

Local autism organizations vary widely in their approaches, so research their leadership, mission, and programming before engaging.

Crisis and Emergency Support

Crisis Text Line provides 24/7 text-based crisis support that can be more accessible than phone-based services for autistic individuals.

National Suicide Prevention Lifeline offers crisis support, though their staff may not have specific autism training.

Local disability rights organizations often provide advocacy support during crises involving discrimination or access issues.

Appendix C: Scripts and Templates

Having prepared language for common situations reduces the executive function demands and anxiety of important conversations. These templates provide starting points that you can modify based on your specific circumstances and communication style.

Disclosure Conversation Templates

Workplace Disclosure to Supervisor

"I'd like to schedule a brief meeting to discuss something that might help me be more effective in my role. I was recently diagnosed with autism, and I've learned some things about how I work best that could benefit our team's productivity.

I want to emphasize that this doesn't change my ability to do my job well—in fact, understanding my autism helps explain some of my strengths, like my attention to detail and ability to focus deeply on complex problems. However, there are a few small accommodations that would help me perform at my best.

Specifically, I work most effectively when I can [use noise-canceling headphones during focused work / have advance notice for meeting agenda items / work in a less visually distracting area]. These modifications would help me contribute more effectively to our team goals.

I'm happy to discuss this further and answer any questions you might have. I've also prepared some information about autism in the workplace if that would be helpful."

Family Disclosure Script

"I have something important to share with you that I've recently learned about myself. After working with a healthcare provider, I've been diagnosed with autism. I know this might be surprising because autism in women often looks different from what people typically expect.

This diagnosis actually explains a lot about my experiences throughout my life—like why I've always been sensitive to noise and crowds, why I prefer detailed planning over spontaneous activities, and why I sometimes need time alone to recharge after social situations.

I want you to know that I'm still the same person you've always known. This diagnosis just gives us a better understanding of how my brain works and what I need to feel comfortable and function well.

I'm sharing this because I care about our relationship and want you to understand me better. There might be times when I need to request small accommodations during family gatherings or ask for understanding when certain situations feel overwhelming for me.

Do you have any questions about what this means or how it might affect our family interactions?"

Medical Provider Disclosure

"I'd like to inform you that I'm autistic, and this affects how I experience and communicate about my health. I was diagnosed [recently/X years ago] and have learned that autism can impact medical care in several ways.

I process information better when I have advance notice about procedures and detailed explanations of what to expect. I also have sensory sensitivities that might affect my comfort during examinations—specifically [light sensitivity/sound sensitivity/touch sensitivity].

Could we discuss some accommodations that would help me be a better patient? For example, [dimmed lighting/advance warning before physical contact/written instructions for complex treatment plans] would significantly improve my experience and cooperation during medical care.

I've brought some information about autism in women and how it can affect healthcare experiences. I'm happy to answer questions and work with you to ensure I receive appropriate care."

Friend Disclosure Approach

"I wanted to share something with you because our friendship means a lot to me. I recently learned that I'm autistic, which explains some things about how I experience social situations and the world in general.

This doesn't change who I am, but it helps me understand why I sometimes need to leave social events early, why I prefer making plans in advance, or why certain environments feel overwhelming to me.

I'm telling you this because I value our friendship and want to be authentic with you. Sometimes I might need to ask for small accommodations, like choosing quieter restaurants or having advance notice about social plans.

I hope this helps you understand me better, and I'm happy to answer any questions you might have about what autism means for me personally."

Dating Disclosure Template

"I'd like to share something important about myself because I feel comfortable with you and want to be honest in our relationship. I'm autistic, which affects how I experience and interact with the world.

For me, this means I sometimes need advance notice for plans, I have sensitivities to certain environments, and I might communicate more directly than some people expect. I also have intense interests that I love sharing with people who matter to me.

I'm telling you this because I care about where our relationship is going and want you to understand who I am authentically. This isn't something that needs to be 'fixed' or changed—it's just part of how my brain works.

I'm happy to answer any questions you have and discuss what this means for how we interact and spend time together."

Accommodation Request Letters

Workplace Accommodation Request

[Date]

[Supervisor/HR Name] [Company Name] [Address]

Dear [Name],

I am writing to request reasonable accommodations under the Americans with Disabilities Act to help me perform my job more effectively. I have autism spectrum disorder, which affects my sensory processing and executive function in ways that can be easily accommodated with minor workplace modifications.

Requested Accommodations:

1. **Noise reduction support:** Permission to use noise-canceling headphones during focused work periods to minimize auditory distractions that affect my concentration and productivity.

2. **Lighting modification:** Access to adjustable desk lighting or permission to position my workspace away from fluorescent overhead lights, which cause sensory discomfort that affects my ability to focus.

3. **Meeting preparation:** Advance access to meeting agendas and materials when possible, allowing me to prepare effectively and contribute more meaningfully to discussions.

4. **Communication preferences:** Option to receive complex instructions or feedback in writing when possible, as I process written information more accurately than verbal information in noisy environments.

Business Benefits: These accommodations will improve my productivity, accuracy, and ability to contribute effectively to team goals. My attention to detail and deep focus abilities are significant assets to our organization when supported by appropriate environmental conditions.

I am happy to discuss these requests further and provide additional documentation if needed. Thank you for your consideration of these accommodations.

Sincerely, [Your Name]

Educational Accommodation Request

[Date]

[Disability Services Office] [Institution Name] [Address]

Dear Disability Services Team,

I am requesting academic accommodations for autism spectrum disorder, which affects my sensory processing, executive function, and social communication in educational environments.

Requested Accommodations:

1. **Testing accommodations:** Extended time for exams and permission to take tests in quiet, low-distraction environments to accommodate sensory sensitivities and processing differences.

2. **Assignment accommodations:** Advance access to syllabi and assignment details when possible, allowing me to plan and organize my work effectively given executive function differences.

3. **Classroom accommodations:** Preferred seating away from high-traffic areas and permission to use discrete sensory tools like fidget items or noise-reducing earplugs during lectures.

4. **Communication accommodations:** Access to lecture notes or recordings when available, as auditory processing challenges can affect my ability to take comprehensive notes during fast-paced presentations.

Documentation: I have attached documentation from my healthcare provider confirming my diagnosis and the need for these educational accommodations.

I am committed to academic success and believe these accommodations will allow me to demonstrate my capabilities effectively while managing autism-related challenges.

Thank you for your consideration.

Sincerely, [Your Name]

Housing Accommodation Request

[Date]

[Housing Authority/Landlord Name] [Address]

Dear [Name],

I am writing to request reasonable accommodations for my disability under the Fair Housing Act. I have autism spectrum disorder, which creates specific housing needs that can be addressed through minor modifications.

Requested Accommodations:

1. **Noise considerations:** Permission to install additional soundproofing materials or use of carpet/rugs to reduce noise transmission, as noise sensitivity significantly affects my ability to rest and function in my home.

2. **Lighting modifications:** Permission to modify lighting fixtures to reduce fluorescent lighting, which causes sensory discomfort and affects my daily functioning.

3. **Service animal accommodation:** [If applicable] Permission for my psychiatric service animal, which provides essential support for managing autism-related anxiety and sensory overwhelm.

Medical Necessity: These accommodations are necessary for me to use and enjoy my housing equally. My healthcare provider has documented that these modifications directly address disability-related needs.

I am happy to discuss these requests and provide additional documentation as needed. Thank you for working with me to ensure equal access to housing.

Sincerely, [Your Name]

Medical Appointment Preparation Guides

Pre-Appointment Preparation Checklist

Two Weeks Before Appointment:

- Research the healthcare provider's office layout and parking options
- Request appointment during your optimal energy time if possible
- Ask about sensory accommodations available (lighting, noise levels, wait times)
- Prepare list of current medications, supplements, and their dosages
- Gather relevant medical records and previous test results

One Week Before Appointment:

- Prepare written list of symptoms, concerns, and questions
- Research your conditions and potential treatment options

- Identify specific examples of how symptoms affect your daily functioning

- Prepare brief explanation of your autism and how it affects medical care

- Arrange transportation that minimizes sensory stress

Day of Appointment:

- Bring noise-canceling headphones for waiting area

- Wear comfortable clothing that accommodates potential examination needs

- Bring fidget tools or comfort items for regulation

- Arrive early but ask to wait in car if waiting room is overwhelming

- Bring written information to share with provider if needed

Information to Communicate to Provider:

"I'm autistic, which affects how I experience medical care. I process information better when I have detailed explanations of procedures beforehand. I have sensory sensitivities to [bright lights/unexpected touch/loud sounds] that might affect my comfort during examination.

My main concerns today are: [list top 3 concerns with specific examples]

My current symptoms include: [detailed description with timeline]

These symptoms affect my daily life by: [specific functional impacts]

I've tried the following treatments: [list with results]

My questions about treatment options are: [prepared list]

I would prefer to receive instructions in writing when possible because I process written information more accurately than verbal instructions."

Post-Appointment Follow-Up:

- Request written summary of visit and treatment recommendations

- Clarify any unclear instructions before leaving

- Schedule follow-up appointments before leaving office

- Ask for written instructions for any procedures or medication changes

- Confirm preferred communication method for test results or questions

Self-Advocacy Scripts

Requesting Sensory Accommodations

"I have sensory processing differences that affect my ability to [focus/participate/function effectively] in this environment. Could we discuss some minor modifications that would help me participate fully?

Specifically, [the lighting/noise level/seating arrangement] makes it difficult for me to [concentrate/hear clearly/remain comfortable]. Would it be possible to [adjust the lighting/reduce background noise/choose a different location] for our meeting?

These accommodations help me contribute more effectively and don't affect others' experience. I'm happy to suggest specific solutions that work for everyone."

Declining Inappropriate Suggestions

"I appreciate your concern, but autism isn't something that needs to be cured or fixed. It's a neurological difference that affects how I process information and experience the world.

What would be most helpful is understanding and accommodating my specific needs rather than trying to change how my brain works. I'm happy to explain what supports actually help me function effectively."

Requesting Processing Time

"I need a few moments to think about this before responding. I process complex information more accurately when I have time to consider it carefully rather than responding immediately.

Could we schedule a follow-up conversation [tomorrow/next week] so I can give you a thoughtful response? Alternatively, would you be able to send me the details in writing so I can review them and get back to you?"

Setting Communication Boundaries

"I communicate most effectively through [written communication/scheduled conversations/direct discussion]. Could we [email about this/set up a specific time to talk/address this directly] rather than [discussing it casually/handling it through multiple brief conversations]?

This approach helps me provide more accurate information and participate more effectively in problem-solving."

Advocating for Different Approaches

"The standard approach to this situation doesn't work well for how my brain processes information. Could we explore alternative methods that might be more effective?

I learn/work/function better when [specific conditions]. Would it be possible to modify the approach to include [specific accommodations]? This would help me participate more successfully while achieving the same goals."

Appendix D: Emergency Strategies

Crisis situations require immediate, practical strategies that you can implement when overwhelmed, overloaded, or facing autism-related emergencies. These tools should be readily accessible and simple enough to use when your cognitive resources are compromised.

Meltdown Management Plans

Early Warning Recognition

Identifying pre-meltdown signs allows intervention before reaching crisis point. Your early warning system might include physical sensations like muscle tension, increased heart rate, or restlessness. Emotional signs often involve increased irritability, difficulty making decisions, or feeling everything is too much. Cognitive indicators include trouble concentrating, forgetting simple tasks, or processing information more slowly than usual.

Environmental triggers that commonly precede meltdowns include accumulated sensory input throughout the day, unexpected changes to routines or plans, social demands that exceed your current capacity, or combination of multiple stressors occurring simultaneously. Recognizing these patterns helps you implement prevention strategies before reaching overwhelming crisis points.

Immediate Response Protocol

When you recognize early warning signs, implement your emergency plan immediately rather than trying to push through increasing overwhelm.

Step 1: Remove or Reduce Input

- Leave the overwhelming environment if possible

- Put on noise-canceling headphones or earplugs

- Dim lights or close your eyes

- Ask others to stop talking or give you space

- Turn off electronic devices or notifications

Step 2: Find Safe Space

- Go to your bedroom, car, or other quiet location

- Use a bathroom stall if no other private space is available

- Step outside for fresh air and reduced stimulation

- Find a corner or less populated area if you can't leave entirely

Step 3: Use Regulation Tools

- Apply deep pressure through weighted blankets, tight hugs, or compression clothing

- Engage in familiar stimming behaviors that help you self-regulate

- Use breathing techniques or count slowly to provide cognitive structure

- Hold comfort items that provide sensory or emotional regulation

Step 4: Communicate Your Needs

- Use prepared phrases like "I need a few minutes" or "I'm overwhelmed right now"

- Text trusted people instead of trying to explain verbally if speech is difficult

- Use gesture or written communication if verbal communication feels impossible

- Ask for specific help like "Please turn off the music" or "I need to leave now"

During Meltdown Support

If prevention strategies don't work and you reach meltdown, focus on safety and minimizing additional overwhelm rather than stopping the meltdown entirely.

Safety First:

- Ensure you're in a safe location away from traffic, stairs, or other hazards

- Remove or avoid sharp objects if you engage in self-injurious behaviors

- Ask others to maintain distance but stay nearby for safety monitoring

- Avoid restraint or physical contact unless you specifically request it

Minimize Additional Input:

- Reduce all unnecessary sensory input in your environment

- Ask others to speak quietly or remain silent

- Maintain consistent, predictable presence without demanding interaction

- Avoid time pressure or demands for immediate responses

Allow Natural Recovery:

- Accept that meltdowns have natural durations that can't be rushed
- Focus on staying safe rather than ending the meltdown quickly
- Use familiar self-soothing behaviors without judgment
- Allow emotional expression without trying to control or stop it

Post-Meltdown Recovery

Recovery after meltdowns requires time, patience, and specific strategies that help you return to baseline functioning gradually.

Immediate Recovery (First Hour):

- Rest in low-stimulation environment with minimal demands
- Engage in familiar, comforting activities that require little cognitive effort
- Maintain hydration and basic physical needs without forcing complex nutrition
- Use sensory tools that typically help you feel regulated and calm

Extended Recovery (Following Day):

- Reduce optional commitments and social demands

- Maintain routine activities that provide structure without overwhelming demands

- Practice extra self-compassion about your need for recovery time

- Monitor for continued overwhelm and adjust activities accordingly

Pattern Analysis:

- Document what triggered the meltdown when you're able to reflect

- Identify which prevention strategies might have helped if implemented earlier

- Note which recovery strategies were most effective for future reference

- Adjust your early warning system based on new patterns you notice

Sensory Overwhelm Emergency Kit

Portable Kit Contents

Create a small bag or container that you can carry with you containing essential sensory regulation tools for emergency use.

Auditory Tools:

- Small noise-canceling headphones or high-quality earplugs

- Smartphone with downloaded calming sounds, music, or white noise apps

- Small portable speaker for playing regulating sounds when headphones aren't sufficient

- Voice recorder for documenting experiences when writing feels impossible

Visual Tools:

- Sunglasses for reducing visual overwhelm from bright lights

- Eye mask for blocking visual input entirely when needed

- Small flashlight for providing preferred lighting in dark environments

- Colored overlays or filters for reading or computer work

Tactile Tools:

- Fidget items that provide preferred sensory input without drawing attention

- Small comfort item like soft fabric, stress ball, or textured object

- Hand lotion or lip balm for self-soothing through familiar scents and textures

- Small towel or cloth for wiping hands if you encounter uncomfortable textures

Regulation Tools:

- Essential oils in small containers for olfactory regulation (if scents help you)

- Glucose tablets or preferred snacks for blood sugar regulation during stress

- Water bottle to maintain hydration during overwhelming periods

- Medications like pain relievers if sensory overwhelm triggers headaches

Communication Tools:

- Pre-written cards explaining your needs like "I am overwhelmed and need space"

- Emergency contact information for people who understand your needs

- Medical information card explaining autism and your specific sensory sensitivities

- Smartphone with text-to-speech apps if verbal communication becomes difficult

Home Emergency Kit

Immediate Comfort Station: Create a designated area in your home where you can retreat during sensory overwhelm with everything you need within reach.

- Weighted blanket or compression items for deep pressure regulation

- Noise-canceling headphones connected to calming audio sources

- Dimmable lighting or blackout options for visual comfort

- Comfortable seating that supports your preferred body positioning

- Collection of comfort items, fidgets, and sensory tools

- Water and simple snacks that don't require preparation

- Preferred temperature control through fans, heaters, or blankets

Environment Modification Tools:

- Extra noise-reducing materials like pillows, blankets, or sound panels

- Lighting alternatives including lamps, candles, or colored bulbs

- Air purification or scent control for olfactory regulation

- Organization tools for maintaining visual calm in your space

Communication Support:

- Pre-written notes explaining your situation for family members or emergency contacts

- Timer or calendar for tracking how long you've been overwhelmed

- Journal or recording device for documenting triggers and effective strategies

- Emergency contact list with people who understand autism and your specific needs

Crisis Communication Templates

Text Message Templates

For times when verbal communication feels impossible but you need to communicate your situation to others.

"I'm having a sensory overload crisis right now. I need [specific request like quiet space/dimmed lights/time alone]. Please don't ask questions right now. I'll explain later when I'm able."

"Meltdown happening. Safe but overwhelmed. Need [time/space/specific accommodation]. Will contact you when I can function again."

"Can't talk right now. Autism-related overwhelm. Please [specific request]. Thanks for understanding."

"Emergency sensory situation. Need to leave/stop/change [specific situation]. Not personal. Will explain when able."

Email Templates for Professional Situations

Subject: Need Brief Accommodation Due to Medical Situation

"I'm experiencing a temporary medical situation that requires me to [modify my schedule/work from home/request deadline extension]. This is related to a documented disability and should resolve within [timeframe].

I will [specific plan for handling responsibilities]. Please let me know if you need any clarification about coverage for my responsibilities during this time.

222

Thank you for your understanding."

Family Communication Script

"I'm having an autism-related crisis right now that makes normal communication very difficult. This isn't about anything anyone did wrong - it's a neurological response to accumulated stress/sensory input.

What I need right now: [specific requests] What would make things worse: [specific things to avoid] How long this usually lasts: [timeframe] How you can help: [specific actions]

I'll let you know when I'm able to discuss this more. Thank you for giving me the space I need to recover."

Medical Emergency Communication

For Emergency Room or Urgent Care:

"I am autistic and currently experiencing [sensory overload/meltdown/shutdown]. This affects my ability to communicate normally and increases my sensitivity to lights, sounds, and touch.

Medical concerns: [list any physical symptoms or injuries] Accommodations needed: [dim lights/quiet room/minimal verbal questions] Emergency contact: [name and number of person who understands your autism] Current medications: [list]

I may have difficulty answering questions or following complex instructions right now, but this will improve as the episode resolves."

Support Person Contact Lists

Primary Emergency Contacts

Contact 1: [Name and relationship]

- Phone: [number]
- Text preference: [yes/no]
- Best times to contact: [timeframes]
- What they understand about your autism: [brief description]
- How they can help: [specific ways they support you]
- Backup contact if unavailable: [name and number]

Contact 2: [Name and relationship]

- [Same information format]

Professional Support Contacts

Therapist/Counselor:

- Name: [provider name]
- Phone: [number]
- Crisis line: [if available]
- After-hours protocol: [emergency procedures]
- Best way to reach during crisis: [phone/email/portal]

Medical Provider:

- Primary care physician: [name and contact]
- Psychiatrist (if applicable): [name and contact]
- Emergency department that knows your history: [hospital name and location]
- Pharmacy: [name, location, and phone number]

Practical Support Contacts

Transportation:

- Reliable ride services that accommodate disabilities: [names and numbers]

- Family/friends who can provide emergency transportation: [contacts]

- Public transportation disability services: [contact information]

Work/School Support:

- Supervisor/manager who knows about accommodations: [name and contact]

- HR representative familiar with your case: [name and contact]

- Disability services coordinator: [name and contact]

Crisis Hotlines and Professional Services

National Crisis Lines:

- Crisis Text Line: Text HOME to 741741

- National Suicide Prevention Lifeline: 988

- SAMHSA National Helpline: 1-800-662-4357

Autism-Specific Resources:

- Autism Society Crisis Line: [if available in your area]

- Local disability crisis services: [contact information]

- Autism advocacy organizations with crisis support: [contacts]

Communication Instructions for Support People

What to Say:

- "I'm here to help. What do you need right now?"

- "You're safe. We'll figure this out together."

- "Take all the time you need. No pressure."

What Not to Say:

- "Calm down" or "Just relax"

- "Why didn't you ask for help sooner?"

- "This isn't that big of a deal"

- Questions about why you're overwhelmed

How to Help:

- Follow your specific instructions without questioning them

- Reduce sensory input in the environment

- Handle practical needs like calling work or rescheduling appointments

- Stay calm and predictable in their own behavior

- Advocate for your needs with other people or in medical situations

Emergency Action Plan for Support People

1. **Ensure immediate safety** - remove from dangerous situations

2. **Reduce overwhelming input** - lights, sounds, demands for interaction

3. **Follow the person's emergency plan** - don't improvise unless necessary

4. **Contact professional help** if safety is at risk or situation doesn't improve

5. **Document the situation** for future prevention and pattern recognition

A Foundation for Managing Crisis

Having comprehensive emergency strategies doesn't prevent all autism-related crises, but it significantly improves your ability to manage overwhelming situations while maintaining safety and dignity. These tools become more effective with practice, so familiarize yourself with these strategies during calm periods rather than trying to learn them during crises.

Your emergency plans should evolve based on your experiences and changing life circumstances. Regular review and practice of these strategies helps ensure they remain current and accessible when you need them most. Share these plans with trusted support people so they understand how to help effectively during difficult periods.

The goal isn't to eliminate meltdowns, sensory overload, or autism-related crises entirely—it's to manage them safely while minimizing their impact on your life and wellbeing. Each time you successfully navigate a crisis using these strategies, you build confidence in your ability to handle future challenges while living authentically as an autistic woman.

Reference

(1) Gould, J. (2017). Towards understanding the under-recognition of girls and women on the autism spectrum. *Autism*, 21(6), 703-705.

(2) Dean, M., Harwood, R., & Kasari, C. (2017). The art of camouflage: Gender differences in the social behaviors of girls and boys with autism spectrum disorder. *Autism*, 21(6), 678-689.

(3) Mowery, M., Haley, M., & Mullaney, R. (2020). Females with autism spectrum disorder: An exploration of autism characteristics and health care utilization. *Research in Autism Spectrum Disorders*, 76, 101-115.

(4) Mandy, W., Chilvers, R., Chowdhury, U., Salter, G., Seigal, A., & Skuse, D. (2012). Sex differences in autism spectrum disorder: Evidence from a large sample of children and adolescents. *Journal of Autism and Developmental Disorders*, 42(7), 1304-1313.

(5) Rynkiewicz, A., Schuller, B., Marchi, E., Piana, S., Camurri, A., Lassalle, A., & Baron-Cohen, S. (2016). An investigation of the 'female camouflage effect' in autism using a computerized ADOS-2 and a test of sex/gender differences. *Molecular Autism*, 7, 10.

(6) Attwood, T., Grandin, T., Bolick, T., Faherty, C., Iland, L., Myers, J. M., ... & Wrobel, M. (2006). *Asperger's and girls*. Future Horizons.

(7) Hull, L., Petrides, K. V., Allison, C., Smith, P., Baron-Cohen, S., Lai, M. C., & Mandy, W. (2017). "Putting on my best normal": Social camouflaging in adults with autism

spectrum conditions. *Journal of Autism and Developmental Disorders*, 47(8), 2519-2534.

(8) Raymaker, D. M., Teo, A. R., Steckler, N. A., Lentz, B., Scharer, M., Delos Santos, A., ... & Nicolaidis, C. (2020). "Having all of your internal resources exhausted beyond measure and being left with no clean-up crew": Defining autistic burnout. *Autism in Adulthood*, 2(2), 132-143.

(9) Howlin, P. (2021). Adults with autism: Changes in understanding since DSM-111. *Journal of Autism and Developmental Disorders*, 51(12), 4291-4308.

(10) Baron-Cohen, S., Wheelwright, S., Skinner, R., Martin, J., & Clubley, E. (2001). The autism-spectrum quotient (AQ): Evidence from Asperger syndrome/high-functioning autism, males and females, scientists and mathematicians. *Journal of Autism and Developmental Disorders*, 31(1), 5-17.

(11) Hull, L., Mandy, W., Lai, M. C., Baron-Cohen, S., Allison, C., Smith, P., & Petrides, K. V. (2019). Development and validation of the camouflaging autistic traits questionnaire (CAT-Q). *Journal of Autism and Developmental Disorders*, 49(3), 819-833.

(12) Chapman, R. (2020). The reality of autism: On the metaphysics of disorder and diversity. *Philosophical Studies*, 177(12), 3575-3592.

(13) Hendrickx, S. (2015). *Women and girls with autism spectrum disorder: Understanding life experiences from early childhood to old age*. Jessica Kingsley Publishers.

(14) Crane, L., Adams, F., Harper, G., Welch, J., & Pellicano, E. (2019). 'Something needs to change': Mental health

experiences of young autistic adults in England. *Autism*, 23(2), 477-493.

(15) Richdale, A. L., & Prior, M. R. (1995). The sleep/wake rhythm in children with autism. *European Child & Adolescent Psychiatry*, 4(3), 175-186.

(16) Lord, C., Rutter, M., DiLavore, P. C., Risi, S., Gotham, K., & Bishop, S. (2012). *Autism diagnostic observation schedule: ADOS-2*. Western Psychological Services.

(17) Happé, F., & Frith, U. (2014). Annual research review: Towards a developmental neuroscience of autism spectrum disorder. *Journal of Child Psychology and Psychiatry*, 55(6), 553-557.

(18) American Psychiatric Association. (2013). *Diagnostic and statistical manual of mental disorders* (5th ed.). American Psychiatric Publishing.

(19) Lai, M. C., & Baron-Cohen, S. (2015). Identifying the lost generation of adults with autism spectrum conditions. *The Lancet Psychiatry*, 2(11), 1013-1027.

(20) Hollocks, M. J., Lerh, J. W., Magiati, I., Meiser-Stedman, R., & Brugha, T. S. (2019). Anxiety and depression in adults with autism spectrum disorder: A systematic review and meta-analysis. *Psychological Medicine*, 49(4), 559-572.

(21) Rucklidge, J. J. (2010). Gender differences in attention-deficit/hyperactivity disorder. *Psychiatric Clinics of North America*, 33(2), 357-373.

(22) Lewis, L. F. (2016). Realizing a diagnosis of autism spectrum disorder as an adult. *Journal of Obstetric, Gynecologic & Neonatal Nursing*, 45(4), 550-561.

(23) Rose, K. (2021). *The autistic survival guide to therapy*. Jessica Kingsley Publishers.

(24) Sedgewick, F., Hill, V., Yates, R., Pickering, L., & Pellicano, E. (2016). Gender differences in the social motivation and friendship experiences of autistic and non-autistic adolescents. *Journal of Autism and Developmental Disorders*, 46(4), 1297-1306.

(25) Sinclair, J. (2013). Why I dislike "person first" language. *Autonomy, the Critical Journal of Interdisciplinary Autism Studies*, 1(2), 1-3.

(26) Hull, L., Mandy, W., Lai, M. C., Baron-Cohen, S., Allison, C., Smith, P., & Petrides, K. V. (2019). Development and validation of the camouflaging autistic traits questionnaire (CAT-Q). *Journal of Autism and Developmental Disorders*, 49(3), 819-833.

(27) Rood, J. A., Rood, T. M., Millenet, S., Lassale, A., Poumeyreau, M., Rosier, A., ... & Chabane, N. (2017). Characteristics of camouflaging in autism spectrum disorder: A systematic review. *Clinical Child and Family Psychology Review*, 20(4), 475-494.

(28) Cage, E., & Troxell-Whitman, Z. (2019). Understanding the reasons, contexts and costs of camouflaging for autistic adults. *Journal of Autism and Developmental Disorders*, 49(5), 1899-1911.

(29) Cassidy, S., Bradley, P., Robinson, J., Allison, C., McHugh, M., & Baron-Cohen, S. (2014). Suicidal ideation and suicide plans or attempts in adults with Asperger's syndrome attending a specialist diagnostic clinic: A clinical cohort study. *The Lancet Psychiatry*, 1(2), 142-147.

(30) Raymaker, D. M., Teo, A. R., Steckler, N. A., Lentz, B., Scharer, M., Delos Santos, A., ... & Nicolaidis, C. (2020). "Having all of your internal resources exhausted beyond measure and being left with no clean-up crew": Defining autistic burnout. *Autism in Adulthood*, 2(2), 132-143.

(31) Robertson, A. E., & Simmons, D. R. (2013). The relationship between sensory sensitivity and autistic traits in the general population. *Journal of Autism and Developmental Disorders*, 43(4), 775-784.

(32) Demetriou, E. A., Lampit, A., Quintana, D. S., Naismith, S. L., Song, Y. J. C., Pye, J. E., ... & Guastella, A. J. (2018). Autism spectrum disorders: A meta-analysis of executive function. *Molecular Psychiatry*, 23(5), 1198-1204.

(33) Gravino, A. (2013). *Sexuality and safety with tom and ellie*. Jessica Kingsley Publishers.

(34) Sutton, M., Webster, A. A., & Westerveld, M. F. (2019). A systematic review of school-based interventions targeting social communication behaviors for students with autism. *Autism*, 23(2), 274-286.

(35) Rothschild, C., & Koenig, K. (2019). Social communication and language characteristics associated with high quality friendships among adolescents with autism spectrum disorder. *Journal of Speech, Language, and Hearing Research*, 62(3), 861-873.

(36) Cassidy, S., Bradley, L., Shaw, R., & Baron-Cohen, S. (2018). Risk markers for suicidality in autistic adults. *Molecular Autism*, 9(1), 42.

(37) Yergeau, M. (2018). *Authoring autism: On rhetoric and neurological queerness*. Duke University Press.

(38) Ne'eman, A. (2010). The future (and the past) of autism advocacy, or why the neurodiversity movement is a civil rights movement. *Disability Studies Quarterly*, 30(1).

www.ingramcontent.com/pod-product-compliance
Lightning Source LLC
Chambersburg PA
CBHW062216270326
41930CB00009B/1751